I'M SORRY
Jimmy Muscle

I'M SORRY
Jimmy Muscle

WHY MY SON WITH
AUTISM WANDERS

DEBRA J. O'FEE

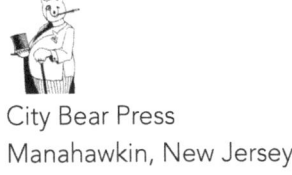

City Bear Press
Manahawkin, New Jersey

Cover image: photo of Ry at the age of 7 by Debra O'Fee
Cover and book design by Lynn Else

Song lyrics on the dedication page are written by Christopher DeGarmo
for "Silent Lucidity" by Queensrÿche © 1990 Sony/ATV Music Publishing
LLC.

Library of Congress Control Number: 2020920373

ISBN 978-1-7351631-1-6 (paperback)
ISBN 978-1-7351631-2-3 (e-book)

Published by City Bear Press
19 Henry Drive
Manahawkin, NJ 08050
www.citybearpress.com

Printed and bound in the
United States of America

To my sons, Ryder and TJ

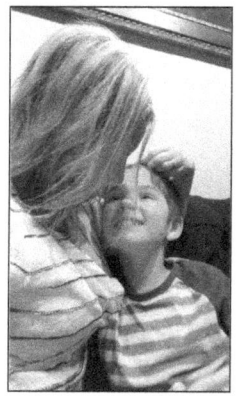

"I am smiling next to you, in silent lucidity"
—Queensrÿche

Contents

Acknowledgements

I would like to thank Louis Conte, for all of the attention he gave me through phone calls, emails, and strategy sessions. He introduced me to the publishing world, and I couldn't have asked for a better coach. I wish nothing but the best for Lou and his family.

Andy McCabe, for his belief that this was an important story that people would appreciate reading. He helped me take it over the finish line to the book shelf. I would like to thank him for his work in the autism community. How can we fail when we have educators like Dr. McCabe in our corner?

Patti Manzi, my editor (I still love those two words), for helping me work through my need to overexplain those highly emotionally fraught topics. Thanks for writing, "Enough. You've made your point—this paragraph is gone! Move on." I really wish I could use some of her "editing" skills in my personal life's dealings!

Every teacher, therapist, and specialist in my school district, including Jennie S., Elizabeth G., Pamela G., Elizabeth S., Catherine C., Kristen C., Eileen P., Veronica F., Laura H., Rachel B., and Jordan M. Thank you, also, to those I have hired privately and who are in my home regularly to work with Ryder, including: Karrie L., Rebecca F., Victoria R. from

Autism Behavior Consulting (ABC); the Com Habs: Michele T., Cassie S., Nadine T., Nicolette H., Bevin S.; and Ryder's "barber," Jackie T. I thank all of them for their kindness to my child and to all of us, especially TJ, my other wonderful son. Knowing that even though he is not the subject of your work, he is a child, too, who needs just as much attention and love as Ryder.

My friends, Louise L. and Theresa Z., who were among the first friends I shared this dream with and encouraged me from the start.

Chief John Aresta and all the Officers in the Malverne Police Department.

My colleagues and friends at Uniondale High School, especially Natacha B., Phil B., Alisa B., Kristine L., and Katie C.

My neighbors, Jerry and Cynthia P., along with Alan and Andrea S., who keep a vigilant eye on our children, as well as my friends at Quality Services Autism Community (QSAC) support group, and my fellow autism moms: Chris P., Julie B., Meredith M., Alison A., Kristen C., and Donna S.

My special soccer friends: Eileen G., Jennifer B., Terry M., and, of course, Kevin F.

My Aunt Diana, Uncle Drew, Aunt Debbie, and Uncle Gary.

My besties: Valerie, Esther, Kristine, and Pattie (even though I know you can't help out in my day-to-day life, I know you have always cheered for me from afar).

My good friends and best neighbors, Lisa C. and Jackie T., and Fran I. for being there *always* and doing carpool duty and for taking TJ to and from religion and also many times taking him along with your own families to functions and events that I could not attend because they would not have been good for Ryder.

The world's best squad ever: Elizabeth, Christopher, Kaitlyn, and Annie for being wise beyond your years and being inclusive and patient with your little friend who loves you all so much.

My mother-in-law, my very best cheerleader, who *only* has encouraging words for me.

My brother-in-law, Chris, whose generosity knows *no* bounds.

My brothers-in-law, Mike and John, and their wives, Debbie and Norma for your constant support.

My brother, Eddie (Muffin), for all the "spectrumy" prep he provided growing up.

Most importantly, a very special heartfelt thanks to my parents for their endless love and support, and for selflessly giving up their retirement to help us. The boys are better for having you in their lives.

Finally, I acknowledge the ongoing support of:

My core group of autism moms, who inspire me daily, especially the moms from Ry's class: Jennifer C., Kim D., Linda F., Maria F., Mary M., and Pam R.

My husband, who I can count on as sure as I can count on Sunday following Saturday— for the times you've shelved a bad day of yours to make way for mine.

My son, TJ, for teaching me about unconditional love, not only by talking-the-talk but by walking-the-walk and walking it absolutely fearlessly *every single day.*

And of course, my son, Ryder, for changing me. I like myself so much better now! You will always be an inspiration and you will always be my little love bug.

Introduction

"God, give me anything, but please don't give me that!"

These were words I uttered in reference to having a difficult child. I was that person—the one who would sneer and tsk-tsk when in the company of a misbehaving child. I was that woman who said with conviction, "When I have children, they will not behave like that!" Then my aunt and uncle had a son, my cousin, Andrew, who was diagnosed with autism. They were always exhausted dealing with the challenges of their son. I developed a different feeling about autism: fear. Autism was now in my family. I started seriously praying, "Dear God, please don't let me be saddled with that when I have my children."

Fast forward. My son, Ryder, was diagnosed with autism.

In trying to navigate all the issues that came up with Ryder, I would reach out to my aunt to ask her about Andrew's childhood. She couldn't remember when certain things happened with him, so I decided to keep a journal. In reading and reflecting on that day's events, I would sometimes laugh, sometimes cry, but I always found what I was reading—what I had just lived hours earlier—fascinating.

Throughout my life, people have encouraged me to write a book, either because of my highly animated way of telling a story or because my stories relate to everyday people. This book is not instructional; most times I don't know what the hell I'm doing with this kid. I didn't study autism formally. I allowed Ryder's school district professionals to counsel me on what's best for him; they are the experts. I often relied on young professionals in their 20s and 30s to fill me in on the latest therapies, programs, and approaches to autism. I have mostly let my heart and my love for this child, combined with a mother's instinct, guide me.

This book is about a person being handed her worst fear in life and living with it. She is not only living with it, but working to overcome it daily; the fear and insecurity never really ends. Does it seem completely unreasonable that I had an overwhelming fear of having a child with autism? In retrospect, yes. Did I ever claim to be a reasonable person? No, not once on these pages will you find that claim.

Growing up, it mattered to me what people thought of me. I worried about my social status, whether or not I was popular. To achieve popularity, I concentrated on how I looked, what I wore, where I went, who I saw—such wasted energy and emotion! Those worries are now a concern of the past. They have been replaced by contentment and peace. I have one person to thank for this; my son, Ryder. I thank him regularly. I thank him for saving me…from myself.*

* Please note that some names in this book have been changed to protect the person's privacy.

1

I'M SORRY, **Jimmy Muscle**

In Maspeth, where I grew up, there was a boy named Jimmy. All the kids called him *Jimmy Muscle*. He was dark-skinned, maybe Hispanic, and a little chubby. He was probably a few years older than me, so when I was 12, he was 14 or 15. He would bop along, always on his own, looking up at the sky, in his own world, and always smiling a kind, harmless smile. He was called *Jimmy Muscle* because he would often offer his flexed muscle for people to feel; then he would ask if he could feel their muscle. He'd say, almost painfully slowly, "Caaan I feeel your muscle?"

Thinking back to the 1980's, I don't remember hearing clinical diagnoses of Jimmy's behavior. People said, "He's slow," or more vaguely and definitely more hurtfully, "There's something wrong with him!" I didn't hear the word *autism* until Rain Man was released in 1988. Today, I believe Jimmy had autism. I'd like to claim that, while the other kids made fun of him to his face by imitating his slow speech, I would jump to his defense and tell them to leave Jimmy alone. But I would be lying. Even worse, when Jimmy approached me to ask if he could feel *my* muscle, I used to scream and run away from him. He didn't realize that the other kids were making fun of him, but he knew by my reaction that I wanted nothing to do with him. And maybe, because of the age, I used to let out an exaggerated scream and run; probably to get more attention from the boys. I was never fearful of Jimmy—you just couldn't be. Jimmy was the gentlest soul that ever walked the earth. His smile was filled with absolute kindness. Even while the other kids were making fun of him, he kept that big smile on his face. When I'd scream, I can remember not so much an expression of much hurt on his face as confusion. *How could she not want to feel my muscle? It's so much fun?*

My son, Ryder, was diagnosed with autism. I can't tell you how often I think of Jimmy Muscle when I watch Ryder. Jimmy Muscle had a sort of hop/skip combo to his walk; Ryder has a similar walk. They also share a special look; their eyes have a sparkle. As with Jimmy, Ryder looks off into the distance, always with wonderment, as if telepathically communicating with spiritual beings.

Jimmy haunts me. I want to go back in time and do the right thing. I want to reverse my behavior and stand up to the other kids and say, "Hey, he doesn't know that you're making fun of him, but I do. Leave him alone!" I try to assuage the guilt by saying that it didn't matter because he didn't understand, he wasn't in on the joke; he was happy.

Every once in a while, I'll pull Ryder closer and I will hug and kiss him and I will whisper, "I'm sorry, Jimmy Muscle."

2

IT'S A BOY! – Again

On January 28, 2010, I was blessed with the birth of my second baby boy. All my life, I had wanted to have a girl and there I was, 15 minutes away from a tubal ligation; the declaration of "It's a boy" meant that the dream of having a daughter was over. My husband and I needed to name our new son and were choosing between the names *Ryder Edward* and *Daniel Edward*—Edward after my dad. At the last minute I couldn't decide, so I let Steve, Stephen, choose between the two. "I like Ryder Edward," he said. And so Ryder was officially named.

Ryder was pretty perfect, I must say. When his brother and grandparents came into the recovery room to meet him, it was love at first sight. Shortly after the visits, a nurse took Ryder to the nursery; she came back to my room and said that she noticed something she didn't like about Ryder's breathing. He was taken to the NICU for observation. Ryder was put into an incubator; he was given oxygen, to be on the safe side. The next morning, a doctor said that Ryder needed a chest tube; there was paperwork for me to sign. I was groggy and tired and I said, "My husband is on his way; he'll take care of that when he gets here."

The doctor was serious and emphatic, "I don't think you understand. Ryder's lung has collapsed; this is an emergency." I signed the paper.

By the time Stephen got to the hospital, I was frantic. And I was in love with my little boy. Ryder stayed in the hospital for eight days, released on that year's Super Bowl Sunday, wearing a Jets' jersey. Thank God, Ryder was fine.

Not only was I no longer disappointed that I didn't have a daughter, I was super-pumped that I had two boys. What could be better? They were close in age: TJ was only 21 months older. The boys could share clothes, toys, friends, and play together. They would be best men in each other's wedding.

But I am getting ahead of myself. Ryder's birth came after a difficult pregnancy. A much easier and successful pregnancy with TJ came after four miscarriages, which doctors believe were due to a blood clotting disorder. Therefore, for both pregnancies, I was on daily blood-thinner injections and regular blood tests. As soon as the *plus* sign appeared during my pregnancy with Ryder, thirteen weeks of nausea, nightly leg cramps, and difficulty breathing followed. I was diagnosed with diabetes, which meant more pricks to test my sugar after every meal. Constipation was so bad that one day Steve had to leave work early to take care of TJ while I sat in the bathroom, fully naked, looking like a Buddha and begging God to let me go. Things did not get better. One week before the scheduled birth, I came down with a stomach virus, got dehydrated, and had to be hospitalized. And, during my pregnancy with Ryder, the country was in fear of a swine flu epidemic. People were dying. Pregnant women, in particular, were most susceptible to the virus. A swine flu vaccine was released, and it was recommended that I have the injection.

I have a cousin who has autism. My aunt is outspoken about the dangers of vaccines. Also, I've always had an unnatural fear of having a kid with autism. This is not to say that I believe any shots or vaccines cause autism, but naturally, I was not crazy about getting injected with something that felt like it had been rushed to market. I had my aunt's warning ringing in my ears. I went back and forth: get the vaccine; don't get it. Finally, I decided to get the shot because TJ's pediatrician, who was at the same stage in her pregnancy as I was in mine, got it. I figured she was in the medical field, she does research, if it's good enough for her, its good enough for me. And then I put it out of my head forever…or so I thought.

3

SOMETHING'S UP **with Ryder**

Ryder was in good health when he came home from the hospital. However, when he was 28 days old, he woke up in the middle of the night with a low-grade fever. I called Ryder's doctor, who advised me to take Ryder to the ER. It was about two in the morning; Steve stayed with TJ while I rushed Ryder to the hospital. His temperature was 100.7. "With anything over a 100.4," a doctor informed me, "we recommend a spinal tap to rule things out."

When I called Steve to share the information, he said that he didn't feel comfortable with a spinal tap; after all, Ryder's temperature was only .3 above the recommended high.

At first, I agreed with Steve, but when I told the doctor that both my husband and I were uncomfortable with moving forward with a spinal tap on our young son, the doctor said, "That's fine, but we need to let you know that a spinal tap is our recommendation." It was said in a way that scared me. I was tired, upset, and fearful that something could be seriously wrong with Ryder. What would happen if we didn't go ahead with the spinal tap and rule out any possible scary things? Or, more importantly, rule them in and start treating them?

I relented and agreed to the spinal tap against Steve's opposition. The doctor suggested that I not be present during the procedure, so I sat outside the room feeling sick to my stomach.

I called Steve. "I told you not to let them do that to him."

I cried.

When the procedure was completed and I was permitted to see him, Ryder seemed fine. He was asleep, in fact.

Ryder and I went home the next morning after the doctors checked him. His fever cleared up later in the day. The spinal tap revealed that he did not have any of the scary things rattled off to me in the ER. I was treated to a big "I told you so," from Steve.

When I told my mother about it, she said, "Steve was right, you shouldn't have allowed that. Cousin Donna refused it, and her baby was fine." I just wonder, where are the people who are supportive, or at the very least quiet, if they have nothing supportive to say? Or are we all surrounded by people who rejoice in telling us how much we screwed up? And for me, it's usually always during a time when I'm already beating myself up. But I digress.

Ryder was the most agreeable baby. Very, very happy; an easy, breezy, go-with-the-flow baby. After breakfast, Ryder would continue to sit in his high chair for a long period of time, never squirming to get out. We lived on the seventh floor of an apartment building at the time, and his high chair was set near the door of our screened balcony. He'd look down at the people below, up at planes, or out at an occasional bird, and he would be content. I would use the quiet time to deal with TJ, or clean the kitchen, or do something a mother of two boys under the age of 3 would do when one child is entertained and secured. When Ryder did raise his arms to be picked up, I could sprinkle a few Cheerios on his tray or put a toy down, and he would remain absorbed for another half hour. This is in no way an exaggeration. TJ was a good baby as well, so when a friend witnessed Ryder being so self-content, she said, "I can't believe you have two such good little boys!"

Early summer, before Ryder was 2, we found a house that we loved in Nassau; this would be a huge move for us. Steve and I had lived in the city our whole lives and I, for the last 10 years, in a high-rise apartment building. Our new house was in a beautiful suburb of homes with lawns and driveways and gardens. Luckily, the owner's daughter was getting married over the summer so we both agreed to a September closing date. We were in rent control, so we were in no real hurry. September would be great; I would have more time to pack, and TJ would still be able to start nursery school in Nassau.

Steve worked full-time so I did all the packing up. I would have to do the brunt of it during the boys' two-hour nap—and that was only when they went down at the same time or when TJ went down at all; he was starting to grow out of them. It was an exhausting process. They say buying a house and moving is one of the most stressful things you can do in your life—I would argue that also having two toddlers makes it even more so.

One day while Steve was home and we were both sorting and packing, he said that he noticed Ryder wasn't talking as much as he used to. I said, "He doesn't talk at all. As soon as we get settled, I'll look into having him evaluated."

I was okay with him not talking because around that age it seemed that every parent of young kids was worried about what their kids were saying—or not saying. Parents of kids Ryder's age would regularly comment, "I don't think my son is saying what he should be at this point." I'm the type who is determined not to get crazy when I see crazy around me. The doctor had asked me about Ryder's milestones. I had told him, and he didn't seem concerned, so neither was I. I did not want to compare him to where TJ was at the same age or to where my friends' kids were at the same age.

When we moved to Nassau, as promised, I made an appointment to have Ryder evaluated.

4

DARK DAYS *of Diagnosis*

Having Ryder evaluated included visits from psychologists and speech therapists. Specialists observed him and interacted with him. They put toy animals on the floor in front of him, and said, "Ryder, give me the giraffe." They asked him questions and monitored his responses.

Ryder didn't do well during the evaluation and was approved for speech services. I didn't ask many questions, but Steve would push for information, and perhaps to confirm his own belief that Ryder was OK, asked the psychologist, "Well, do you think it's anything more than delayed speech?" Information was not forthcoming.

I would try to rationalize the position of the therapist to Steve by insisting that no one could tell us too much after only a short evaluation. We argued. I look back and wonder how Steve could have thought that he would be given answers so quickly; he looks back and how I could have been in denial. It's not that I was trying to delay the diagnosis; it's that I felt a thorough diagnosis would take time. The psychologist who completed the evaluations was a man named Dr. Adam Vance. He was warm and patient with Ryder and with Steve as well. He was not at all condescending, which was something I feared he would be the minute I read the "PhD" on his card. Admittedly, I am easily intimidated by people whom I believe are more knowledgeable than I am. Dr. Vance, however, was reassuring in his demeanor and approach.

Ryder was given two half-hour sessions each week with a speech therapist, to whom he responded very well. His first speech therapist was Michelle, a 50-something woman, who managed to get Ryder to sit with her and work on the routines that were required for speech therapy. I thought that this, in itself, was a feat. Ryder was not yet 2. When Steve was home, he'd corner Michelle at the end of the session to try to discuss what she thought, "in her experience," was going on with Ryder. Again, we'd argue. I'd say, "Steve, even if she thinks it is autism, she's not going to say it. She's here for the services, not the diagnosis. We have to wait for Dr. Vance."

After six months, Dr. Vance was ready to review the evaluations and lay out a plan for moving forward. Since there was very little improvement in Ryder's speech, as part of the overall plan, Dr. Vance added two sessions of applied behavior analysis (ABA) to the speech therapy each a week.

This began with a woman named Angela. We adored Angela. She was able to have Ryder sit in a chair for 45 minutes and respond to her instructions. Steve tried to discuss Ryder with Angela and, again, aside from going over how Ryder progressed during the session, she did not elaborate on a specific diagnosis. She would say, though, that it *could be* that Ryder had a processing issue and gave us some tips on how to strengthen his progress. Ryder responded to sensory and physical prompts; Angela would hold his hands and have him jump, facing her. Ryder did become responsive to subsequent prompts. When Steve was concerned about Ryder's weak use of direct eye contact, Angela taught us to use a paper towel roll and play a game with Ryder, making him look through the cardboard and focus on our eye, on the other side.

One day during this six-month stretch, Steve again pressed Michelle, and she admitted to him that she thought Ryder could possibly have autism. I shared this with Angela, who disagreed; she did not think Ryder had autism. Steve and I wanted to believe her, but we had our private doubts. We met again with Dr. Vance, who was well-aware of our concerns. Ryder had undergone a full year of speech and ABA services with very little progress. It was impossible to stifle Steve during the meeting. Dr. Vance took a lot of notes during our conversation, but he did not commit to anything specific. He did say that Ryder was stumping him a little bit because "there is plenty about him that is not pointing to autism, Mr. O'Fee."

He told us he would go back to his office, review his data and the reports from the therapists, and call us in a few days with his findings.

On December 21, 2012, a month shy of Ryder's third birthday, Dr. Vance called. Steve and I were on separate phones, listening together. Dr. Vance gave us his diagnosis: PDD–NOS. There it was: autism. PDD-NOS stands for *Pervasive Developmental Disorder–Not Otherwise Specified.*

The thing I most feared, having a child with autism, just happened.

In December 2012, people were emerging from the shock of Superstorm Sandy, our area was hit especially hard, and parents were burying their children following the horrific shooting at Sandy Hook elementary school in Connecticut; at home, my small Long Island family had just received the answer to why our nearly 3-year-old was not progressing "normally." I felt bad, and then I felt bad for feeling bad with all that was going on around me in the world, but I couldn't help myself. I just felt bad.

One day during this fog of sadness, I was driving with both of my sons in the car. A song by the Lumineers came on the radio. TJ said, "I love this song," and started singing, "*I belong with you, you belong with me, you're my sweetheart….*" He sounded so angelic in his young 4-year-old voice. I pulled the car over right there on Grover Avenue and turned around to listen to him sing. When the song ended and TJ was finished singing, Ryder, in the next car seat, started clapping. I believed that God had just given me a sign that everything was going to be OK.

5

MY NEW **Autism Diagnosis**

The thing about autism is that once your child is diagnosed, it often feels as if you're on your own. Educational needs are met by specialists within the school district, but there's no single liaison, social worker, or anyone who says, "OK, here's what you do next." There's no "OK, you have an official diagnosis; here's this person assigned to you for anything you might need to know…" That's what I felt that I needed. The psychologist provided website links on the bottom of the report and encouraged me and Steve to use them as resources. So soon into the diagnosis, none of them seemed to pertain to what we needed…yet.

Working with Ryder turned out to be a *learn as you go* experience for us, which, in retrospect, I'm not so sure may not be the best way to handle a diagnosis like Ryder's. Each child is different; symptoms and behaviors vary widely, and responses to therapies are often inconsistent and unpredictable. I often think that if you were to know out of the gate what you "may" go through, you *may* have a breakdown, right there and then, at the time of diagnosis. In time, your child's needs become apparent, and you learn what to do:

> If he's not learning enough with the approved schooling, call in an outside agency for additional, at-home services.
>
> If your child is an eloper/wanderer, look into tracking devices.
>
> If your child tries to flee the house, get a locksmith to secure your doors and windows.
>
> If your child is petrified of the vacuum, put it in the garage.

The list of symptoms is as long as the list of children with an autism or PDD–NOS diagnosis. There are free, community-based organizations and support groups, but overall, help can be expensive. There are agencies that help with financial aid, but rarely is there someone to tell you how to apply for it right at the point of diagnosis. When you do unravel the process to get such aid, it is not easy to follow all the protocols. The paperwork is often complicated, lengthy, and time-consuming. You know what else is time-consuming? Raising a kid with autism.

Let me share one story about my "learn as you go" experience with financial aid.

My mom found out that there's a Medicaid service designed to help people apply for aid. When I got in touch with the office, I was put in touch with a Medicaid coordinator. Following our conversation, the coordinator left me with quite a few papers to fill out. She told me that, after completing them, I needed to return them to the Social Security office. I didn't get two pages into the sixteen-page packet when I realized I couldn't fill them out: I didn't understand any of it. It was like trying to provide answers in English to questions written in Chinese. I called my Medicaid coordinator and tried to explain that I didn't understand what the questions were asking. She said that she would put me in touch with a non-Medicaid coordinator, who might be more helpful. Dennis, the non-Medicaid coordinator, came to my house to help. He skimmed through the packet and asked, "She wanted you to fill this out yourself?" He actually started to laugh.

I said, "Yes. She said that I needed to take them, completed, to the Social Security office." I was not laughing.

He explained that there were three steps that had to be taken, after the paperwork was finished, before I could go to the Social Security office. He began helping me from that point on. Like everything bureaucratic, the process moves slowly. We did get all sixteen pages filled out over the course of several weeks. I'd like to tell you what the next step is following the return of the paperwork, but after six months, we're still waiting to learn.

6

PARENTS AND OUR
Living Arrangements

When Steve and I talked about making the move to Long Island, we decided to get a "mother/daughter" structure so that my parents could move in with us yet have their separate "apartment." They would be with us to help out with the kids. My parents agreed to the plan, and also agreed to help contribute to paying the bills.

Steve, the boys, and I moved into our new home in September, as I've said. The following November, my dad moved in while renovations on his part of the house were ongoing; my mom stayed in Staten Island until her upcoming retirement in December. Dad returned to Staten Island to be with mom for weekends. By February, renovations were completed and we were settled into our new living arrangement.

Admittedly, Steve and I tend to be disorganized under the best of circumstances. However, with both of us working full-time while trying to manage multiple schedules, house construction, household routines...well, there's bound to be more than the usual disorganization. My dad is generally easy-going. He has a good sense of humor and a willingness to listen and play with the boys. Mom is extremely generous and dependable, if, perhaps, a bit less able to turn a blind eye to chaos. Living with two boys under the age of 3 in a house undergoing construction can certainly test anyone's patience. My parents' tolerance was no exception.

My dad loses his cool when the boys become rambunctious, and I will never meet my mother's standards for "keeping house." Overall, however, we've learned to adjust to one another. I always wanted my parents to have a close relationship with my kids. Grandparents are all about unconditional love and spoiling, right? Of course, once we were all living together, the spoiling often gave way to some disciplining. I appreciate some of the very special things that occur between my children and my parents. TJ goes to church each week with my mom and says his prayers with her each night. His relationship with my dad is off-the-charts great. They playfully goof on each other and learn from each other, too. TJ has learned so much from my dad and shows sincere love and affection for him. My mom provides unlimited love and care for Ryder. She's absorbed by his progress and is vigilant about his safety. However, despite all these positives, there is a reason why more people don't decide on this co-living arrangement.

Sometimes Steve and I feel as if we're still kids living in our parents' house. My parents inevitably revert to their roles as protectors. "Are you sure that jacket's warm enough?"

"Mom, I'm 47 years old."

There are some special rituals they share with the boys, though. My Mom and Ry go to the price club together, and he loves it. He's so good with helping load and unload the car; the routine makes him feel helpful and responsible. My

Dad, TJ, and I have a standing appointment to watch certain TV shows together, including *The Big Bang* and *Young Sheldon*. As TJ has been getting more homework, my Dad has been helping him with his school assignments. I'm convinced he's the only 75-year-old who knows Common Core math.

Some of Steve's and my friends question our sanity. I am sure my parents sometimes question their own sanity when they agreed to take on this new post-retirement living arrangement.

As I mentioned, I will never be the housekeeper that my mother is. Let's face it, dealing with Ryder and the special attention he needs would challenge the most domestic of the goddesses. Once, I remember, Steve's family was coming over to spend some time with us. After I cleaned the house and straightened up, my mom said, "I saw dust underneath the couch."

I looked. I didn't see it. I said, "Mom, my child has autism." This, to provide perspective as well as commentary on how unimportant hard-to-find dust under the couch is. Her response was, "Oh don't blame him. He didn't put the dust there."

I must say that things have improved over the three years that we've been together. We've worked out most of the kinks; the ones that recur are settled with a therapeutic blow-out once or twice a year. Steve and I have the luxury of having loving, dependable, live-in care for our boys and my parents have the luxury of having time and purpose with their grandsons. The boys keep them busy and sharp, that's for sure! Perhaps down the road, we will disband and my parents will be able to enjoy a different retirement of socializing with peers, bingo, and golf, but for now, we're good. We're great.

7

SCHOOL **Meetings**

Pervasive Development Disorder–Not Otherwise Specified (PDD–NOS) is also known as Autism Spectrum. As ridiculous as it sounds now, I thought the word *spectrum* meant *sprinklings* of autism or *outer edges* of autism. I did not understand it to mean, *full-blown* autism. I perceived *spectrum* to mean *characteristics slightly similar to someone with autism*. Clearly, I had a lot to learn. Once we received Ryder's diagnosis, we met with school district counselors. Ryder was diagnosed in December 2012, and in January 2013 we had our first meeting, the first time I had a meeting at school when I wasn't the student. So, twenty years after just managing to finish high school and spending a year at a community college before realizing that I was more of a worker than a student, here I was about to enter a school meeting. I felt like a fraud; like someone playing grown-up.

Everyone at the meeting was extremely supportive, sensitive to the fact that my son had literally just been diagnosed with autism. No one mentioned the diagnosis or the word *autism* during the meeting. They told me we were eligible for more services in the home—more hours of Michelle and Angela—or part-time schooling out of the house. Ryder was a boy who liked being around people, not that he interacted with them, but he liked being around them. Knowing this about Ryder, and knowing that my parents needed downtime from the boys, Steve and I opted for the out-of-home school provision. Until Ryder was accepted into a school, services at home would be increased.

The school district sent information about Ryder to area schools so that they could consider his eligibility for their programs. In the meantime, Angela, who knew how badly we wanted to get Ryder into a school, put feelers out. She found there was a spot in the school operated by ACDS (formerly, Associated Children with Down Syndrome). Once known as a Down syndrome school, it incorporated, some time ago, an autism program to accommodate the growing number of children with PDD–NOS and autism diagnoses. Ryder was accepted into their school. Ryder adjusted well. He seemed to enjoy getting out of the house and being at school.

By the end of the school year at ACDS, we did not see much improvement: it was time to take things to the next level. At the urging of my aunt, I brought Ryder to see a neurologist. I thought that he was a rather gruff, too unemotional man for the role he had. After evaluating Ryder, he said in a rote tone, "I'm looking at moderate autism in this child."

I said, "He was diagnosed with PDD."

"Your child has moderate autism, not PDD."

I said, "I'm sorry, I studied up on the statistics for PDD and 38% of PDD children lose the diagnosis in childhood. By age 17, how many children with autism lose the diagnosis, Doctor?"

He looked at me and said, "Mrs. O'Fee, he's not losing this diagnosis; your child will always be autistic."

My heart sank.

I think I understand now why I misunderstood that PDD and autism were two different things. Autism is one of many things that come under the PDD umbrella. Specialists hesitate to immediately come out and say *autism* because they're not really sure about the diagnosis when they evaluate children who are young. Kids learn on different timelines; maybe the child is slower, but not really autistic. PDD really means, *We still have no clear idea what's going on with this kid so here's an umbrella diagnosis to allow for future specificity and some immediate services.* This gives parents who are desperate for answers something to go on. We wanted answers, and now we had one. It was time to get Ryder into a school program that would accommodate his needs.

I have some gripes with school meetings and goals and testing, although I have respect and admiration for the people with whom we've worked in our district. New York State uses test scores that pool Ryder, and children with different learning issues, with "typical" learners in the same grade. It is disheartening to hear, in meeting after meeting, that Ryder's test scores are in the 1 percent bracket for his age or that his reading level is "below average." How about letting me know how he is measuring up to other kids his age with learning disabilities or create a different measuring system. A helpful tip someone gave me is that I should not measure Ryder against any kid other than the Ryder of six months earlier. It would be nice if the State did the same.

Fortunately, Ryder was a good fit for the 8-1-4 setting offered by our school district: 8 kids, 1 teacher, and 4 aides. I use the word, "fortunately," because my district currently does not have programs to accommodate all the children with the varying levels and manifestations of autism. When a child is unable to fit into one of the current curriculums within the district, parents have to send that child to a school that specializes in their child's disability. This has caused frustration and often anxiety for some of the parents with children with special needs in my community. I know from my autism support group, comprised of parents with children with autism from Nassau and Suffolk counties, that there are many school districts that do not have in-district programs to accommodate their children.

On the one hand, I'm happy because the school program in my district has worked out for Ryder; on the other hand, I am aware of my fellow "special needs" parents' frustrations and struggles. I have come to understand how a district might not be able to accommodate all levels of autism—it *is* a broad spectrum. I read recently that one in 54 children have an autism diagnosis today. It seems that as far as we've come in our progress in identifying and treating and educating children with autism, we still have a long way to go. I would like to see more expansive programs in the schools across all districts.

8

WE HAVE **an Eloper**

A few months after we moved to Long Island, I was playing on the back deck with both boys. TJ asked me to help him assemble his train tracks; I became absorbed in lining and connecting the tracks with him. After a while, I stood up and noticed that Ryder wasn't in the yard where he had been playing moments before. I went inside the house to look for him and saw that although the front screen door was shut, the inner storm door was open.

I rushed outside to look for Ryder but didn't see him. I assumed that I had panicked unnecessarily, so I went back inside and moved from room to room to look for him. No Ryder. With anxiety rising, I reached the very last unsearched room; when I didn't find him there, I raced back to the front door. My heart was pounding. The moment I stepped outside, I saw my new neighbor, Jerry, strolling up my walkway with my not-quite-two-year-old son in his arms.

Once Ryder was gently handed over to me, I collapsed in tears of relief right there on the stoop. Jerry tried his best to console me, but I couldn't speak coherently enough to thank this man for his kindness.

Later, when I spoke to my parents and with some friends to share the day's unexpected upheaval, each advised me not to tell Steve. After all, things turned out OK, it was probably "one of those things" that happen with kids, why upset Steve?

Two days later, the boys were playing with two neighborhood girls. The kids were racing around the house playing some version of tag or hide-and-seek. They were loud, the groceries needed to be put away, the mailman was at the door, the phone was ringing...the usual chaos of a household with kids.

At some point, I looked up from organizing a snack for the gang and saw TJ with the two girls—but no Ryder. *Oh my God, where's Ryder?* I barely choked out the words as I ran up the stairs to look for him. There he was, in his room, playing on the floor with a toy truck. I sagged against the door frame.

TJ and the two girls, sensing some excitement might be afoot, had followed me upstairs. One of the little girls looked at me and said innocently, "Did you get so scared because the other day Ryder got out and Mr. Peterman found him almost around the block?"

The word was out: the new family couldn't keep track of their kids. The next morning, I told Steve all that had happened. We shared a new understanding: Ryder acted on his own impulses to play by himself or to wander off to explore the world. We had to watch him differently than we did TJ.

Even after multiple discussions with Steve and with my parents about the need to keep Ryder under careful watch, it happened again: Ryder escaped. I was sitting on the couch going through some bills in front of our bay window. I knew that Steve was with TJ or my mom was with Ryder or vice versa. I happened to look up and saw my 2-year-old strolling down the street without a care, completely on his own, as if this was exactly what he was allowed to do. As I rushed out the door to gather Ryder into my arms, I yelled back to Steve and my mom, "How hard is it to keep a 2-year-old inside the house?!"

This was not the end.

The absolute scariest elopement was on May 14, 2015. My dad was on double-duty coverage with TJ and Ryder, bridging the time between after school and my return from work at 5:30 in the afternoon. My dad mentioned that morning that he was concerned about helping TJ with his homework while trying to keep an eagle-eye on Ryder. If I could go back in time, I would have said right there and then, "Leave the homework to me."

But I have to admit, I wanted the luxury of having TJ's homework finished before I got home, so I didn't speak up. I will forever regret it.

I called the house about 4 pm as a routine check on things. As soon as my dad answered the phone and heard my voice, he blurted, without even a *hello*, "Ryder got out."

I told him to relax and to look inside the shed in the backyard. Ryder often went there when he wandered from the house, and I felt there was a good chance my dad would find him inside playing with one of the stored seasonal decorations. "I'll stay on the line, dad," I said. "Take the phone with you and let me know when you see Ryder."

I listened as my dad, with the cordless phone, walked outside and opened the door to the shed. "He's not here, Deb. And the side gate is open." My heart jumped into my throat. "Dad, go look for him. I have to call 911."

Our house is in the center of a seven-house block: three houses to the right is one corner, and three to the left is another corner with a busier street. If Ryder turned one of the corners and my dad chose to go in the opposite direction, Ryder would have even more time to get farther away. I called 911 and explained, through rising panic, that my nonverbal, autistic son was missing from my house in Nassau County; I was more than 20 minutes away in West Babylon. While precious seconds passed, my call was transferred to the appropriate jurisdiction. I had to repeat that I was calling from West Babylon and that my nonverbal, autistic son was missing from my home in Nassau County. I was screaming the information that they requested: his name, his age, his height, and what he was wearing. I knew it all. I told them he was wearing his yellow and gray *world's most awesome brother T-shirt.*

I had raced out of my office and was weaving in and out of traffic, hoping a cop would stop me; I wanted more help. The 911 responder let me know that police cars were en route to the area where Ryder was last seen.

Barely able to control myself, I called my dad to see if Ryder had returned. He had not. I heard TJ in the background crying and asking, "Pop-Pop, what if a stranger gets him?"

And then my mind raced to all the horrible things that might befall my baby: he could be hit by a car, lost in the nearby woods, injured by a fall, and of course, picked up by a stranger.

I remember my dad telling me to calm down while I was driving. Calm down? This is my baby, the boy who was not aware of the dangers of traffic or water or strangers. I hung up the phone. And then dad called back. "Deb, he's home."

Never had I been so relieved.

When I arrived, there were three police cars in front of my house, lights flashing. An officer opened my car door

and said, "Don't worry, Mama, he's home safe and sound…
it's OK."

I said, "It's not OK." I choked and violently vomited
right there, all over my front lawn.

I ran up the three front steps into the house and saw
Ryder on the floor, playing peacefully with his big brother.

The police officer who drove Ryder home told me that
a woman, driving with her daughter, saw Ryder wandering down the street near her home. She got out of the car
when she saw police cars and waved them down. The police
brought Ryder home. TJ, relieved to have his brother home,
was, of course jealous of the ride in a police car.

It was time to heed the advice given on the National
Autism Association's website. I sent a flyer with Ryder's picture to each of my neighbors. It let them know that Ryder
has autism and that he is an eloper; it requested that,
should they see him alone on the street, to please call me
immediately, and if possible, to gently bring Ryder back to
our home. The flyer included my name, address, and phone
number.

Not ten minutes after delivering the flyers, Bart, an
older man who lives up the block, called me. He said that
he and his wife were sitting out earlier in the day and saw
Ryder walk by their home. They assumed someone had an
eye on him or that he was allowed to walk around the block;
he looked happy, not lost or confused. Bart and his wife
live on the corner of our street three doors from my house.
Our nightmare could have been avoided right then had the
couple known to call me or to stop Ryder.

The National Autism Association's website recommended I go to my local precinct to put on record that
Ryder was an eloper. So, I did.

Once there, I told the officer at the desk that my son
is non-verbal. He has autism, and that he tends to wander

and bolt. The officer was completely perplexed. He asked me to wait while he went in search of information; he did not know what I was talking about. Or why. He returned with information from someone at the precinct who knew about this. Basically, if a 911 call comes from my house, the police who will respond to the call get a message from the dispatcher that, although it may or may not be related or relevant to the specifics of the call, there is a young boy with autism who lives at the address. Police with this knowledge will respond to the call with autism protocols in mind.

While I was there, I told the officer about what had happened earlier in the week. I explained that there was a woman in the car with Ryder when he was rescued and returned home. I wanted to thank her if I could, since in all the upset of the event, I let her slip away, unacknowledged. The officer explained that since everything was resolved within 20 minutes, no official report was filed, and therefore, they had no information about the woman. He, however, knew that the officer who answered the call dropped the woman back at her home and possibly had an address. That officer was off duty on the day I was at the precinct; the desk officer would call me when his colleague returned to work. The officer who rescued Ryder called me the next day and told me that he dropped the lady off at the corner of Gems Lane. He also gave me a few more details: she stayed with Ryder after she hailed the police car; once the police stopped, she remained with Ryder while he was driven home because he seemed calm while she was with him and more unsettled when she tried to leave. Her daughter drove their car back to their house.

Gems Lane has a lot of houses and I decided not to go door-to-door looking for the woman who took the time to care for Ryder and see that he was returned home safely. I do think of her as my Gems Lane angel, though, and hope that by sharing her story here, someone else may be inspired to look twice and act responsibly if he or she sees a child walking alone.

I took the story of Ryder's escape to my local mom's group. I was afraid that when I told my story, someone would respond saying, "*You need to watch your kid, Lady.*" Instead, I received helpful feedback, support, and more information regarding the incident. One woman told me that she saw what happened when the police cars arrived. "Ryder tried to take off when all the cops showed up," she said. "It was funny watching him and them. They didn't know how to catch him with people starting to gather and watch, I guess."

I'm assuming that the police didn't want to try to grab him for fear of hurting or scaring him. Unfortunately, Ryder's really like a frisky puppy when he gets out and people attempt to catch him: he takes off running. He's that way with Steve and me, too.

I feel that each time I say a specific problem related to autism is *the absolute worst*, it's as if Ryder hears me, takes it as a challenge, one-ups me, and shows me something worse. So, while I used to feel that eloping was worse, I've since realized that no, it's not. Bolting is.

Bolting is worse than wandering because wandering can be reasonably controlled with watchfulness. I do my best never ever to let Ryder out of my sight. But the bolting comes out of nowhere, even when Ryder's within inches of me. It's random, it's fast, wild, and there's no control over it. So, I do believe that, while he's wandering, he mostly follows a route and some rules, as if he were walking with us, staying on the sidewalk for example. If a car approaches, sometimes Ryder will stop. The bolting is another thing. Ryder becomes so preoccupied with getting away as fast as he can that he might dart onto a busy road with no regard for oncoming traffic.

I take Ryder and TJ to "special soccer" on Tuesday nights at the local elementary school. All the kid's in Ryder's class are there with their siblings. The kids get to run around—the special needs boys and girls usually without focus—while their siblings get to play indoor soccer and socialize. As we all know, gyms and school buildings have multiple entrances and exits as well as designated emergency exits, as they should.

One night, Ryder made a run for the gym's emergency exit. I ran immediately to chase after him. Mind you, I am usually cognizant of the layout of the buildings we're in because I need to be aware of the perimeters and possible hazards. However, it was winter and the program had just started, and I had not found the time to do my usual "walk-through" of the building. I knew the exit led to a playground, but I did not know exactly whether there were steps outside the door or a gate into the playground itself.

When Ryder made his dash through the exit, Kevin, the coach, followed me out the door. I prayed Kevin, who was more fit than I was, would not give up the chase and leave it to me. It had become dark, so I had to slow down in fear of tripping over a step; there would be no catching Ryder with a sprained ankle or broken leg. I picked up speed when I felt the cement change to grass underfoot.

Thankfully, I caught sight of Ryder just ahead. I lunged forward, grabbed him by the back of his shirt, and pinned him to the ground. Ryder laughed happily at what he perceived to be a great big game; I wanted to give him a good old-fashioned spanking. But of course, that would have been both futile and just plain wrong. Instead, I caught my breath, pulled Ryder upright, and gave him a big hug.

Kevin, Ryder, and I walked back inside, trying to maintain a sense of calm and good humor for Ryder's sake.

When I looked back to the escape from the gym that night, I actually thought about some of Ryder's remarkable abilities. His young eyes acclimated to the unlit, dark school yard; it was clear he was not trying to "find his way," as I was. In addition, Ryder was fast! He proved to be quite a runner with both speed and stamina. And for better or worse, he was fearless. Perhaps without worry about possible obstacles, my little one will take risks that will strengthen his learning and social skills.

Anyway, I did return to explore the building, its entrances and exits, its steps and stones and discovered that the schoolyard was completely fenced-in. If only I had known beforehand!

Shortly after that event, I decided to have a fence installed around my yard to enable Ryder to play outside more freely and to provide a safe enclosure whenever he bolts out the back door. I discovered that there are different agencies that help fund home modifications for families of autism children. I worked with a local agency to help defer the cost of the fence. One of the things I had to submit for their consideration was a list of the numerous times Ryder bolted or eloped. Needless to say, the list was long. Writing the list brought to mind one of Ryder's more notable escapades.

My Aunt Diana and Uncle Drew were visiting from Staten Island. My uncle worships the Catholic saint, Padre Pio, a saint of miracles. Our church has a beautiful statue of the saint, so when Uncle Drew visits, my mom takes him to see it.

Whenever family or friends put on their coats or shoes, Ryder understands that they're "getting out" and he wants to go with them. Late one afternoon, there was really no reason for Aunt Diana and Uncle Drew not to take Ryder along to visit Padre Pio. After all, my mom and dad would also be with them, too, so Ryder was under the watchful eyes of four adults. As the group stood in front of the religious statue, praying for Ryder to outgrow his bolting and eloping tendencies, Ryder bolted off into the darkness behind the statue. There they were, my three sexagenarian relatives, prayers left unanswered, chasing Ryder in the dark recess behind the statue of Padre Pio. Luckily, they retrieved him rather quickly—or so they told me.

Ryder remained blissfully unaware of the level of worry that he created that day. The worry was surpassed, as it always is, by the level of love that is felt for him.

9

ACTIONLAND – **Part 1**

The first time I realized that outings with Ryder could range from uneventful to downright life-threatening was when he was 3-years-old and TJ was 5. On a breezy summer night, Steve and I took the boys to Actionland, an O'Fee favorite destination.

Actionland is a little amusement park a few miles from the house. It's perfect—reasonably priced and never over-crowded. It's always a fun time. At age 3, Ryder's autism was not necessarily visible. For example, a 3-year-old is not always chatty, so no one would notice that Ryder wasn't speaking as he should be.

The boys were on and off a few rides, having fun. There were no long lines, so because he didn't have to wait, Ryder—along with the rest of us—was spared a meltdown. We were all having a solid, bona fide, good time.

Then I put the boys on a car ride which circles a track with a maximum height of fifteen feet, reached at a point directly opposite the starting point. So, if you're facing it, the track looks like an O that's falling slightly backwards. Since this is a ride that goes extremely slowly and holds the cars on the track from underneath, there are no railings on either side. There's no need for them, really.

The boys were buckled into seats in the same car. Once the cars began moving, parents waved to their kids, calling out names and taking pictures. The ride had music and some strobe-like lighting flashing as the cars went around and around. When the ride came to a stop and the exit gate opened, parents rushed to retrieve their kids. A few moms and dads got ahead of me and blocked the path to my kids. Then I heard some "Oh my Gods" and turned to see Ryder running up the track. I grabbed the confused ride operator, a 16-year-old teenager, and screamed, "Get that kid!"

In movies, when something tragic is happening things seem to go in slow motion and the sound becomes very low and focus is on the person watching the drama unfold… that was what happened to me. I saw Ryder approaching the highest point of the ride, looking wobbly, without rails for support. I saw terror on the young ride operator's face, and a combination of concern and undeniable envy on TJ's face. Everything else was a blur.

While all this happened in a matter of seconds, it certainly felt as if time stood still. As soon as Ryder got close enough, Steve, who had already run up the track, grabbed him and pulled him into his arms. I turned to the ride operator and said, "I'm so sorry, my son has autism." This was the first time I said the word *autism* in reference to my son.

Although the drama was over, there were a few parents and kids lingering, probably waiting for more excitement. One woman came up to me and said, "You know, they have 'special' nights here for children like him."

Today, I can look back and be sure she meant to be helpful. At the time, however, I felt hurt and angry. I found myself wondering and imagining: *What the hell goes on here on those nights? Bunches of spectrum kids hanging from roller coaster structures?*

Having regained my composure, I simply thanked her for the information and walked to join Steve and the boys. I learned something that night: Ryder saw things differently. While most kids understood the rules and restrictions of an amusement park ride, Ryder did not. Ryder wanted to walk on the tracks and saw no reason not to do just that. It would be my job to try to anticipate Ryder's creative perceptions and possible predicaments and to stay one step ahead of him.

10

WATCHING **Ryder**

I have wonderful friends who mean well and have offered to watch my son. They say things like, "I don't take my eyes off my kids; I won't take my eyes off Ryder."

Actually, most parents believe that they don't take their eyes off their kids, but they do. It's natural. I would—and did—take my eyes off my son until I realized the difference between him and other kids. Ryder has behaviors associated with his diagnosis that require not attentiveness, but vigilance. In a nanosecond, Ryder can seize an opportunity to run, bolt, and cause himself harm.

Once the warm weather hits, Ryder will *not* stay inside after school. In fact, once spring arrives, Ryder *needs* to be outdoors. Let me describe how under ordinary circumstances this would not be a problem but how unordinary the simple agreement, "Sure, you can go outside and play in our fenced-in backyard."

My parents enjoy a weekly bingo game at our local church. The minute I pull into the driveway from work on Thursday afternoons, my mom and dad, with bingo chips and markers in hand, literally rush past me as I approach the front door. Usually, Ryder is with them and is handed off to me as they hurry out.

One day, however, Ryder was not with them. "He's here waiting for you," my dad said as he skipped toward the sidewalk. Something was just a bit off; my parents seemed to be escaping as opposed to just leaving. But it was their bingo day, so I hurried inside.

The instant I walked through the door, I smelled it. Ryder was still wearing diapers—another part of the autism experience I had to accept. Anyway, let me assure you that a 5-year-old's poop, especially if it has been sitting in a diaper, is much more rancid than that of a toddler. Clearly, Ryder needed to be cleaned and changed right away.

The instant I finished changing him, Ryder made a beeline for the back slider doors and ran into the yard. I had to make the dash after him! I had not had time to bag his dirty diaper and discard it nor to wash my hands. I had to be outside with this child *pronto*.

Instead of taking that extra minute or two to clean up as another parent might, I had to hit the backyard only to sit and watch Ryder play. I watched him. He watched me. Ryder was waiting for that moment when I might turn my head or go inside and leave him for a minute, as I used to do before I learned his practices and pranks. So, there I sat for almost an hour while I waited for Steve to get home from work. There I sat, *willing* my hands to be washed and the bathroom cleaned.

Finally, Steve emerged through the sliders. Instead of a smile and a warm welcome home, Steve caught, "Stay here and watch him," as I dashed past him and ran up the stairs. From behind me I heard him say, "I just literally walked in the house! Can't I change out of my work clothes before you pass him off to me?"

At last, able to wash my hands, I thought: *No, Steve, you can't. Like I couldn't toss out the diaper or wipe down the bathroom or wash my hands. Like I can't turn my head any of those times when TJ wants to show me something. Like I can't change my clothes and relax for a few minutes after work before I deal with Ryder.*

That explains why I don't trust even my most treasured friends to take care of Ryder. We had to make adjustments for going out as well as adjustments for staying at home. To ensure that Ryder was under our watch, we would travel out as a family. Otherwise, either my parents, Steve, or I would stay at home with Ryder. Often, Steve and I would go to events separately so that one of us could stay home with Ryder. Steve would go to his family's gatherings and celebrations; I would go to mine. Often, only one of us would be able to go to a friend's event.

These seemed like small sacrifices to make to stave off the worry of Ryder's unpredictability. Many times, we started out as a family when there was a kid's party or game, but if things proved too unmanageable or uncomfortable for Ryder, one of us would leave to bring him back home. We always try to give Ryder as many experiences as we can and risk having to leave an occasion rather than regret that *he would have loved it.* I want people to see him, and I want him to see people and learn to be with them appropriately. If I isolate him, how will that help him? I also discovered that Ryder often provides the perfect excuse to duck out of undesirable events early. Shhh…I did not admit that!

Ryder has taught me to reserve judgment. Things happen with kids, even to the most attentive, loving parents. I read a story about a boy who had special needs and a disorder that manifested in compulsive eating. The boy's parents were learning about his special needs and behaviors. One night, he soiled through his mattress; his dad brought the mattress outside the house and hosed it down. The story also claimed that, because the boy roamed the house at night, a video camera was installed in his bedroom to enable his parents to keep an eye on him. One day, following a minor car accident which left his mother a bit unsettled and which exacerbated the boy's behaviors, he begged for some food in addition to what he had eaten for lunch. His mom gave him some, but not did not allow too much. Soon afterward, the boy became extremely sick. He was rushed to the hospital and eventually died; it was concluded that he died of sodium poisoning. The mother was charged. Evidence of child abuse used against her included the wet mattress, which was still outside, the video surveillance system, and an opened box of bouillon cubes in the pantry.

At one time I would have jumped on the bandwagon of accusation. However, after learning to live with and love Ryder, I fully understand how all the "evidence" could be proof of efforts to watch and care for a child with special needs and how the salt could have been consumed in an instant of momentary distraction.

Apparently, Ryder does not like the scent of perfume. I used to enjoy wearing different scents and had quite a collection of pretty bottles. That is, until I understood Ryder's "game." I think it was his way of letting me know he did not like the smell of flowers or spices on his mom. If he could get his little hands on one of the perfume bottles (in one of my inevitable seconds of distraction), he would hide the bottle but leave the cap for me to discover. At first, when I saw a bottomless cap, the decapitated bottle hopelessly gone from sight, I would rush to Ryder to smell his breath to make sure he had not swallowed the liquid. Relief would sweep over me when he passed the breath test, and I knew that he was OK. But what if just once Ryder *had* tasted the scented liquid? What if I had to rush him to the hospital? What would a stranger think? Would I be judged as a negligent, or worse, abusive parent?

The point is that it's easy to judge or speculate when you haven't walked the proverbial mile. My friend's son, also an eloper, got out of her house one evening in December. Thankfully, a neighbor saw him and called her, but she had already called the police. My friend, Meredith, arrived at the corner where her son was waiting at the same time the cops arrived. The officer who answered the call for help began to question her. Because she was barefoot, her feet were cold and she innocently asked if they could hold the conversation at her home. When she realized her son was out, she took no time to put on shoes before racing outside to look for him. A woman, barefoot on a cold sidewalk in December, relieved her son was found, is not neglectful, but she still has to answer the how's and why's of her son's getaway.

I no longer judge my fellow autism moms and dads. Instead, I pray that my fellow parents have the opportunities to safeguard their children, especially as they become aware of each new potential hazard.

11

MY ADVOCACY **Awakened**

I decided to research personal tracking devices to help keep Ryder safe. Some were too expensive; others seemed too big or too small to be practical. When I came across Project Lifesaver, I remembered hearing about it at my autism support group. Project Lifesaver International is an organization that has developed a protocol for tracking at-risk children and adults. The program uses a radio transmitter that emits a pulse that can be picked up by a local police department. A responder can locate the person wearing the device via the "beeps."

As I continued my search for a tracker for Ryder, I met John Aresta, the chief of a small police department in Malverne, a community that was about a 35-minute drive from our home, and longer with traffic. He supported Project Lifesaver. Chief Aresta gave me the application and told me what I needed to do to qualify for the Lifesaver device. A few months after I filed the necessary papers, Chief Aresta called to inform me that Ryder's Project Lifesaver band was ready. He came to our home to put the transmitter on Ryder and show us how it works. We initially put it on Ryder's wrist. The chief said, "Oh he won't be able to get it off; the wristbands are really sturdy."

After the first day with his wristband, Ryder got off the school bus and carefully placed the transmitter in my father's hand. Ryder seemed pleased that he had removed it himself. The next day, we attached it to his ankle. Ryder left it there, accepting it as a new part of his routine.

I learned that Ryder was the ninth person in Nassau County to get the Lifesaver unit. Chief Aresta and his officers were supporting the growing project throughout Nassau County. I promised I would help garner more support for the program; more responders and scanners were needed. Ideally, the responders should be within five miles of a wrist or ankle band unit.

I began my advocacy with a letter-writing campaign. To strengthen my argument for more extensive Lifesaver support, I shared what I discovered as I read and researched: Today, one in 54 children have autism; this includes one in 45 boys. I learned that 48 percent of people with autism wander. People with autism are attracted to water; 91 percent of accidental deaths of people with autism are caused by drowning. My focus is the autism community, but Lifesaver transmitters are important for other at-risk populations, including adults who suffer with dementia or Alzheimer's disease or Down syndrome.

In addition to sending letters to local and county officials, I spoke with key people throughout the area. While some appeared fully interested in my goals, others seemed polite, but anxious for the conversation to end. I assured each and every one that I was not going away. "I'll be back in touch soon," I said with a smile to each contact. My persistence resulted in success. Project Lifesaver was rolled out and officially supported by the Nassau County Police

Department less than a year after Ryder received his. I can't claim that my efforts alone made this happen, but most people I spoke with in the Nassau County offices knew me, my son, and our story.

My advocacy for Project Lifesaver was inspired by Chief Aresta. He was moved by compassion for autism families although, as he told me, "There is no one specifically who got me going." His initiative in taking on Project Lifesaver program was not easy: there were miles of red tape to cover and countless colleagues across the county to solicit for support. The chief, along with the members of his local department, supported the program themselves for over a year: they filed applications, helped process payments, entered computer data to align with back-up scanners, and dealt with frantic moms of missing kids and caregivers of missing adults. After Chief Aresta had been so patient and helpful to me, how could I not help him?

My advocacy of the Project Lifesaver program had an additional impact on me: it strengthened my voice as an autism mom. I lost all hints of shame or guilt, feelings that are so common among autism parents. I shed my need for privacy. I became a tiger-mom on behalf of other parents, who needed a voice to share information, support, compassion, and optimism—and humor.

12

AUTISM & ALL His Friends

If there's one thing I feel I can boast about, it's that I'm a good friend. I am a loyal, hands-on friend, who does not desert people in times of trouble.

I have one friend who, unfortunately, is doing a stint in jail. Since his crime is one of fraud and one that touched several mutual friends, Aidan has been abandoned. I write to him every month or so even though to date, he's never responded. A response would be welcome, but I'm not writing with the expectation of getting something in return; I'm writing to let him know that he is not alone. There is a degree of isolation that comes with the embrace of Autism that has made me far more sensitive to conscious or unconscious acts of exclusion.

Walter Winchell, a popular journalist through the mid-20th century wrote that, "A friend is someone who walks in when others walk out." I have become a friend to Autism: I remain loyal despite his demands, I am a hands-on advocate for his causes, and I am certainly constant in times of inevitable trouble. Having autism in one's circle, however, is not easy. Autism's dominant personality has alienated many less formidable friends and family members.

Let me be clear: I am no martyr! I am going to tell you right now that I do wallow in the luxurious spa of self-pity every so often. I often yearn for the good-old-days of a carefree girls' night out. I also want some of my "old" friends to offer emotional support, even though the kind of support that an autism mom needs is often incomprehensible to anyone "outside." Sound as if I'm whining? Indulge me! I need to lay just a bit of guilt on anyone of you who knows an autism mom, maybe because you knew her "when" or maybe because you see her at school events, but have abandoned her. Take the time to get to know her! Invite her out for lunch. Send her a note. Smile when you see her – don't run away. Know that beneath all the bravado there is someone who feels overwhelmed (often) and lonely (sometimes).

Remember, too, that Autism is the pal who never leaves her side. He enters her home and usurps her time and her energy. Autism becomes part of her family. I want both my boys to share events with others. I want TJ to enjoy a break from Autism; he needs invitations that give him time with peers away from us. So another call-out: do you know an autism family with a "typical" sibling, one who you might invite to a ball game or sleep-over or movie? The typical sibling often becomes overlooked because the shadow of Autism is ever-present. I urge you to make an effort to include the brothers and sisters of autism children in some of your plans.

I question how to remain a source of comfort to my friends as they deal with the issues that affect them. They deserve a comforting friend. I try to keep Autism in his place and provide support for those around me who need the occasional metaphoric hug. Although I have to confess that

I find it more and more difficult to relate emotionally, and definitely socially, with people with whom I used to be so comfortable. As most close friends and family do, Autism has changed my personality. I used to love a big party! I used to love large gatherings replete with laughter, song, and dance. With Autism as my partner, I've become more withdrawn. Sensory overload causes me to find more comfort in tranquil moments of walking quietly and appreciating my surroundings; this, a complete reversal of how I used to be.

I can't blame my friends for any disconnect, they have not changed; I have. I have undergone a slow morphing into someone different from the person who they've known. Once, a close friend asked, "What happened to you? You used to be so sharp and now you don't seem to understand what I come right out and tell you. You seem to be distracted all the time!"

I responded, "I have autism now".

All is not doom and gloom! There is a flip side to my grumbles. I have added new friends and people with amazing insight and strength into my life. The women in my autism support group have proven to be indescribably supportive and are remarkable sources of available services and specialists. The moms of the other kids in Ryder's class are kindred spirits, willing to share their time and energy with me. There are therapists who walked through my door and taught both me and Ryder skills necessary for physical, emotional, and social growth. Ryder's first teacher, Jennie, has become a treasured friend. Even a former administrator from my school district, who was there for me when I was just beginning to learn the autism game, became a trusted friend, long after she left the district.

My passion is to support my fellow special needs moms. The word is out: I am there for moms of children recently diagnosed. I let these moms know that their circle of friends is bound to change. Autism will test the patience and the endurance of some old friends; there is no doubt about that. However, Autism invites new and often unexpected friends into our lives. To offer the words of one more writer, this time C.S. Lewis, "Friendship is born at that moment when one person says to another, "What! You too? I thought I was the only one."

13

ACTIONLAND – **Part 2**

It was Ryder's pre-school graduation day. We planned, weather permitting, that, after the ceremony, we'd surprise TJ by pulling him out of school and taking both boys to Actionland. After Ryder's moving-up ceremony, Steve, Ryder, and I went home to change out of our dress clothes into play wear. I decided to put on an autism parenting T-shirt that I bought a while back but, until then, had not been ready to wear. I figured that maybe people at the park would see it, and if Ryder were trying to cut the line or something, they would put two and two together and be more understanding.

The weather had been questionable all day with threats of thunderstorms. I called Actionland and learned their policy: if it rains for an extended period while you're there for under three hours, then you get a rain-date pass. It was hard to make it through three full hours with Ryder under the best of circumstances, so with nothing to lose, we picked up TJ and off we went. The skies were grey and the park was empty. Perfect!

The day was going great. The four of us were going on rides in varying combinations: sometimes, Steve or me with the boys; and other times, the two boys together. There were one or two rides for which Ryder was too short and one or two that were too kiddie-ish for TJ. Steve and I were adept: divide and conquer and make each boy happy. Steve opted for some of the kiddie rides (he liked to stand by and watch); I took TJ on the water log after which we emerged soaking wet and smiling.

Several times during the day we walked past an enormous walk-and-ride attraction in the middle of the park. TJ kept bugging us to go through it with him. The pirate-themed amusement involved a walk-through plank path that wound high up to a maze of enclosed slide tunnels and wiggly bridges and twists and turns and all sorts of things that were not visible from the ground below. There were sections of a slide tunnel very high up that looked as if they were not covered or enclosed. Instinctively, I sensed the dangers for Ryder. Once up at the top, Ryder, I vividly imagined, would find a way to pull himself up and over the side and plummet to the ground below. "TJ," I said, "you can't go in there today. It's too dangerous for Ryder." TJ was edging closer to the entrance, my words fading behind him. Steve picked that moment to declare that he was thirsty, and he headed in search of some water.

TJ turned around to face me and repeated, "I want to go on this ride," and moved closer to the entrance. Ryder chimed in, "I go. I GO!"

Defeated, I agreed to go on it with both boys. I laid out a plan, as I always do. "TJ, you get in front. Ry, will stay in between you and me and we'll all walk together."

TJ nodded his agreement and entered the tunnel. In no more than a heartbeat, Ryder overtook him. Ryder scrambled up and over his brother and began his tear through the maze. Weighed down with backpacks, hunched down to fit through the twists of the maze, crawling as fast as I could, I yelled, "TJ! Go after him!"

"Mom, he's right here. Mom, I'm with him."

I breathed a momentary sigh of relief and crawled closer to the boys. The boys continued through the tunnels, over the bridges, and around the twists staying reasonably close together.

I was not too far from them as we neared the last long slide that exited back into the open park. I called to TJ, "Wait and hold Ryder at the top; I can get ahead of him and wait for him at the bottom when he comes down."

"What Mom?" TJ answered as I watched Ryder get into position for his slide out.

I yelled, "Never mind. Go! Just go after him! Get him!"

Ryder went down the slide as fast as a bullet. TJ should have been sliding just as fast to catch up with his brother, but he was not moving. His shorts were still wet from our water ride and there was not enough traction to allow him to slide. Breathless, I caught up with TJ and the two of us, trapped in wet shorts, used our feet and arms to force our way down this slide tunnel. I could see the ride monitors down below. Banging on sides of the slide with all my might, I screamed to the girls in charge, "Stop that little boy!" but heard myself echoing in the enclosure, so I knew they could not hear me. And then I saw Ryder shoot out of the slide and take off into the open park like a Labrador Retriever freed from his leash.

Timing is everything. Just then, Steve returned, bottle of cold water in hand. He spotted Ryder and took off after him. Father and son returned as TJ and I emerged from the tunnel slide. Steve's reaction to finding Ryder on the loose was fast and furious, "What the *hell* were you thinking?!"

Instead of escalating the tension, I knew that the best thing to do was to move on. Usually an incident with Ryder means that he was in some kind of trouble or danger. There is no reason to berate the chaperone, who already feels awful. Steve tends to hold on to the anger underlying his relief when Ryder is again safe.

To put the day back on track and to restore the boys' enjoyment of the attractions, I agreed to let them go on the climbing wall. I checked out the attraction. It was a wall with colorful stepping stones and ropes the boys could use to steady themselves as they climbed. There was an enormous red cushion under the ropes in case of a fall. If worse came to worst, Ryder could just fall onto the cushion. Needless to say, I underestimated Ryder's perspective: I saw a climbing wall; Ryder saw a means to return to the pirate cove from which he had *just* been captured.

No sooner had he begun the climb than he jerked quickly to the left and around to the back of the climbing wall and out of my sight. I will spare you the details of my renewed sense of panic and of the ensuing chase. Finally, though, Ryder was back in my line of sight, heading directly toward the exit of the pirate slide. I took off, determined to grab him before he entered it. I have to admit, I was really hoping some strong 12-year-old would come flying out of the tunnel and knock Ryder down like a bowling pin. I reached Ryder as he entered the bottom of the slide; he had managed to scramble several feet up the tunnel when I, now lying face-down and hunched in the tunnel up to my shoulders, put a death-grip on his ankle.

As I was trying to pull Ryder out, I felt someone trying to help by dragging *me* back out. I felt my back scraping against the roof of the tunnel, and I felt something sharp scratch my back but I was not going to release my grasp of Ryder's ankle. I yelled, "Please! My back is hurt..." It was

Steve, who had come to the rescue. He pulled me, I pulled Ryder, and once again, we were standing upright on *terra firma*. My back was bleeding and in pain; there must've been some nail or metal thing that caught me maybe hanging off the top of the covered slide. I lifted the back of my shirt for Steve to look at how bad it might be and I heard TJ say, "Oh my God, Mom, your bones are out." My bones were not out. It was those white skin scrapings like the ones you got on your knee when you were little. TJ thought they were bone chips.

Steve gently poured some of his water on my lacerated back. Then the four of us sat quietly on a nearby park bench. We had been at Actionland for two-and-a-half hours. It was hot, my shirt was bloody, the boys were tired, but happy. It was time to go. As we were leaving, defeated, TJ said, "Oh Mom, your pretty nice new shirt is ruined." It was then that I looked down at the words on my T-shirt: and as if to mock me, I saw it...the words: "Keep Calm... I'm an Autism Mom."

14

ABOUT **Ryder**

When I cuddle with Ryder I whisper, "I love you just the way you are. I wouldn't change a thing."

"You know when I hear you say that to him," Steve often responds, "it goes right through me. Wouldn't you want him to talk? Wouldn't you want him to be more aware and be able to be more appropriate for his age?"

"Ryder needs to hear the words that match the hug. He's my baby, and I love him just the way he is, Steve."

Ryder doesn't talk much. He doesn't share his feelings or come home to tell me about his day at school. He relays happiness with smiles and laughter, a bad mood with agitation. He lets his dislikes known with protest: a swift loud, "NO!"

If I'm not on site when he gets hurt, I don't know why or how any bruise occurred. At times, I have wondered whether or not he feels physical pain; he doesn't yell or cry when he falls or gets hurt. Sometimes, I'll learn about an injury from the school. One Monday, I got a call: "Mrs. O'Fee, earlier today when we were helping Ryder in the bathroom, we noticed a bruise on his thigh."

I racked my brain but couldn't remember anything that happened over the weekend. I couldn't recall seeing a bruise when I bathed him the night before. When Ryder came home from school that afternoon, I pulled his pants down and there it was: an enormous, ominous-looking bruise. I was still trying to recall the events that might have caused the injury when TJ remembered. "Ryder fell off the top step of the bunk last night after his bath. You heard it from downstairs because it made a loud noise."

TJ was right, but when I ran upstairs to see what happened, Ryder seemed fine. He never cried and barely even winced. By the time I got to him, he was sitting on the floor, playing with some toy trucks.

I usually learn about a loose tooth after I discover a gap in Ryder's smile. Once, one front tooth was obviously loose; I checked each adjacent tooth, but none seemed wiggly. I was ready for the loose one to come out. I double-checked all the teeth before Ryder went to bed that night. He woke up in the morning with two front teeth gone! I called for Steve, who ran upstairs to help me look for the missing teeth. We stripped the bed but found nothing. Ryder probably swallowed the teeth during the night. When Ryder lost a tooth, it was often *lost*. I used to get upset when things like this happened, but I've learned to keep calm, as long as there is no imminent danger. Steve and I were OK, but TJ worried about Ryder missing out on the tooth fairy visit. That crisis was solved when we had TJ draw a picture of Ryder's teeth and the drawing was put under the pillow. The first couple of times that TJ did this, we included a note to explain the situation. "Dear Miss Fairy," the note read,

"Autism stole Ry's tooth again." Now, just the drawn tooth is enough. The tooth fairy gets the drill.

It's also hard to tell if Ryder is coming down with something. He doesn't tell me if his throat hurts or if his belly hurts, like TJ does. Fortunately, both boys are in good health and visits to the pediatrician are infrequent. The lack of general communication such as, "Mom, I have a stomach ache," adds an additional need for heightened observation and care. I often think about some of the basic things we take for granted with typical kids.

Ryder may be uncommunicative, but he is not without personality! He is gentle, sweet, affectionate, playful, and happy. He likes people, even though he doesn't often interact with them. He likes being among people and is at ease in a crowd. Ryder is a hard worker; he will come home from a full day at school and then willingly work with the ABA therapists for another two hours.

There was a time when I worried about whether Ryder felt compassion. Like many children with autism, he seems self-absorbed. Then one day, TJ was crying. Ryder sprang up, ran and got a tissue, and returned to dab TJ's eyes with it. We watched in disbelief. This was such a loving gesture. Most importantly, it showed that Ryder noticed TJ was crying and that he responded appropriately. Actually, Ryder knocked it out of the park response-wise.

Ryder is a little boy who is not fully cognitive of what is going on in the real world around him, the world in which he's supposed to participate and function. He has a pre-occupation with fantasy, and therefore, he has a hard time understanding when he should be attending to his real-life environment. He is so often absorbed by what goes on in his own imagination that he doesn't want to leave it; he is literally living in his own world, which seems to be more seductive than our own. This has caused learning delays.

The children who can be pulled out of their autism worlds have the potential to grow, mature, and function as independent adults. The ones who can't be lured, well, don't progress—at least not by society's standards.

I don't know the point at which parents realize their children won't ever come out of their autism worlds to live independently. Do parents stop therapies when that realization is reached? There are moms in my autism support group who already believe that their kids will never be able to live on their own. I am not there yet in my thinking about Ryder, which, I guess, is a good thing. What is the next step following surrender? I have to trust that decisions will become clear as Ryder and I move forward. Hopefully, if it turns out that he will not reach his potential as a fully-functioning, independent person, the realization will have come so gradually that my heart will be prepared for it.

Ryder does know a lot of words, and he'll respond when I ask him. He's verbal when he needs to be, but he doesn't speak beyond the bare minimum. In fact, Ryder needs to be prompted before he will speak. I have the feeling, autism aside, he's the strong silent type.

Autism has cast a whole new light on discipline. I always thought I would be a hard-ass, strict mom. Not so. In fact, I'm just the opposite; I am there for tickles, cuddles, and hugs. Of course, it's hard to know what, if anything, will work when it comes to disciplining Ryder. There is a distinction between a tantrum and a meltdown and there are distinctions in how to deal with each and its aftermath. A lot of meltdowns occur when Ryder perceives that rules have been changed on him. He can't just roll with the punches. We have learned to narrate to prepare him for the things that are about to occur: sometimes it works; other times it doesn't. For example, we have to talk him through the process of getting a hamburger if the venue is different from the one to which he is accustomed. At All American, the system is that you place your order, get a number for it, back up and wait until your number is called, then return to the window to pick up your order. This is different from McDonalds, where you place an order, wait a few minutes at the counter, and then get the food. The first time Ryder went to All American, he had no understanding of why he heard me order a burger and then step away from the counter, no burger instantly presented. Despite an ongoing explanation of what was happening, Ryder completely lost it! Somehow, he got a grip of the window on the other side of the counter and wouldn't let go. A piercing scream accompanied his iron-clad grip. As I was trying to wrestle him from the window and loosen his hold on the counter, he yelled, "Debbie, No! No, Debbie!" Ryder calls me Debbie, so it appeared to the shocked onlookers that I was an aggressive babysitter rather than a mother who would eventually calm her son. Peace was restored when the burgers appeared.

BounceU is a rental venue for birthday parties and play dates. Our Special Ed group schedules events there during weeks that the kids are on break from school. Birthday parties include pizza and cake after the jumping; play dates do not. I have not left a play date at BounceU without having to calm Ryder, sometimes while he has molded himself to the party room door while yelling, "I want cake!"

You would think that after all this time I could predict what might be next, but *no*, I'm just not creative enough to do that. Once, on our way to our favorite restaurant, I narrated the upcoming sequence to prepare Ryder for the evening: *Ryder will have a hamburger, Ryder will sit like a good boy wherever they seat us, even if it's not Ryder's favorite table. Ryder will have ice cream with whipped cream at the end of dinner if he's a good boy.* Repetition got us from home to inside the restaurant. While we were waiting to be seated, I looked at both my boys, who looked especially adorable. The hostess appeared and told us to follow her; I went first, TJ next, Ryder, and then Steve. We were the picture of a nice-looking, well-mannered family. Then I heard, *"Hey, you can't just take that!"* On our way to our table, Ryder reached out and snagged something off another diner's plate. After that incident, my narration included the instruction not to touch anyone else's food. We learn as we go.

Ryder has slowed me down, heightened my awareness of my surroundings, and strengthened my empathy toward others who struggle—whether with autism or with other challenges. I love to be at the park with Ryder and watch him play. I try to wonder what is going through his mind and imagination. At such times, I pause to appreciate all of Ryder's special qualities and his emerging personality. But I have given up trying to predict his unpredictability. And I wouldn't change a thing.

15

VACUUMS, **Hair Dryers,** **Lawn Mowers**

Applied Behavior Analysis (ABA) is the application of the principles of learning and motivation from Behavior Analysis, and the procedures and technology derived from those principles, to the solution of problems of social significance. Many decades of research have validated treatments based on ABA. For example: Applied Behavior Analysis (ABA) is a therapy based on the science of learning and behavior. ABA therapy applies our understanding of how behavior works to real situations. The goal is to increase behaviors that are helpful and decrease behaviors that are harmful or affect learning (www.autismspeaks.org).

Steve and I decided to add in-house ABA therapy to Ryder's traditional schooling. ABA therapists work to improve communication and social skills and decrease problem behaviors. They design a plan on an individual basis and then practice until mastery of a skill or modification of a behavior is achieved and advancement can take place. Each autism student is unique and responds differently to the various treatments, so initially, strategies are based on some trial and error. Ryder responded to a system that included small rewards for success.

Ryder had a phobia of certain things that make noise, such as a hairdryer, vacuum cleaner, and the electric trimmer used for his haircuts. We had to keep the door to our master bathroom closed with the hair dryer secured behind it to enable Ryder to come into the bedroom without fear. And despite a ceremonial event heralding the removal of the vacuum cleaner from the house and into the garage outside, Ryder wouldn't stay on the main level of the house for almost a year. "Bye-bye vacuum!" Then, in a parade, Steve, Dad, Mom, and TJ, escorted the Hoover out of the house into the garage while Ry and I watched and waved from the upstairs window. Afterward, Ryder would still rush past the closet that had held the vacuum, especially when entering or leaving the house. In fact, his phobia prevented Ryder from eating his meals in the dining room with us because of its proximity to the closet; he ate upstairs in his bedroom. There were two Christmas mornings when Ryder wouldn't stay downstairs to enjoy the frenetic unwrapping of Santa's loot!

The ABA team began by desensitizing Ryder to the hair dryer and the hair trimmer simultaneously. The therapists kept the hair dryer in the room while they worked on an unrelated lesson and in between positive words and smiles, they'd lean over and turn it on. To tame the fear of the trimmer buzzer, they would bring Ryder into the bathroom six to eight times per session, turn it on, and pretend-buzz his hair. To my surprise, Ryder recovered from both fears in a very short time; the vacuum cleaner took longer.

I recall the shift from hatred to love of the once terrifying appliances. One day, following weeks with the ABA therapists, Ryder brought the vacuum cleaner into his play area and stood it among the stuffed animals, dolls, and trucks. At one point, I saw him looking for a plug in which to plug it in so that he could hear the noise! Luckily, he heeded the "no, no" when he was told not to put anything—including the newly adored vacuum cleaner—into the power sockets. Then there was the night I saw him snuggling the hair dryer and falling asleep while cradling it.

I may have made the transition away from fear sound easy. It was not. As I said, the vacuum cleaner recovery took much longer than the recovery from the other appliances. The ABA girls didn't introduce a system to get him over the vacuum fear until they felt confident that his fear of the other two appliances was overcome. I remember the first few days during which they put the vacuum outside of the room in which he was working; it was heartbreaking to listen to his screams. You must have a thick skin to hear your child's absolute terror and not be able to remove the source of the fear immediately. Children with autism do not just grow out of a sensory fear over time like more typical children do. For *months*, the vacuum was taken out of the garage and put right outside his ABA work room. Countless times per session, the therapists would interrupt the regular lesson to open the door and say, "Hi vacuum." Sometimes they would pat it gently as they repeated, "Hi vacuum." Then, one day we heard, "*hi, vacwoom*," followed by heaps of praise from his ABA therapist, Tori. Steve turned to me from where we were perched upstairs and said, "Ryder is hugging the vacuum." Ryder earned praise after praise from us as well as a round of applause when, with a big smile, he took my hand and brought me to meet his new friend, the vacuum.

After Tori left that triumphant afternoon, Ryder wouldn't let us put the vacuum back into the garage. He wheeled it around, tried to unzip the bag, leaned it forward then backward, unwound the cord, and pressed the on/off button over and over again. Steve's friend and his son were doing electrical work that day; very proudly, Ryder took their hands to show them the vacuum cleaner. TJ wasn't home that afternoon; after his religion class, he went to his friend's house for a play date. He returned to witness Ryder's four-year fear of the vacuum cleaner completely reversed. TJ had been home for no more than ten minutes when Ryder casually strutted by wheeling the vacuum cleaner on the main level of the house. TJ looked at the vacuum to Ryder to the vacuum again and then at me, and with a huge smile on his face said, "Ryder's with the vacuum cleaner." I answered, "I know," as if it were the most natural thing in the world.

There were other behavioral and social habits that needed to be addressed. The eloping and bolting remained an immediate concern that took priority. Ryder needed to be able to walk with us, calmly, down the street. We kept Ryder in the stroller longer than he should have been there. After that, we moved him into one of those toddler cars that has a handle at the back of it for pushing and pulling. Ryder's a big kid, so his knees jutting above the steering wheel made him look cartoonish. I needed to be able to walk alongside Ryder, not holding his hand. Our ABA team is helping me. Ryder and I practice walking together, conversing. I say, "We're walking, we're walking nicely," with the hope that he will smile and repeat the words and stay by my side. However, sometimes, BAM! He takes off. My reaction is key. If I chase him and scream—my natural response—Ryder sees it as a game. The therapists have lowered my scream to a loud call, and my own mad dash to a strategic stride. When Ryder is captured, we resume, and in a calm voice, albeit through gritted teeth, I say, "Ryder, we are walking nicely down the street." Yes, it's true: we are going through our own ABA therapy and modifying our behaviors to help Ryder modify his.

Going out to dinner poses its own set of potential problems. Mostly we go to a restaurant called the Corner Galley, two blocks from home. Ryder loves it there. In fact, it's one of the places listed as a check point on his REACH identification card should he go missing. The people there know Ryder and are very accommodating; Ryder likes to sit at one specific table so they try to hold it for us when they know we're coming. Because of its familiarity, things usually go well there.

Our last restaurant experience was at a different restaurant, one unfamiliar to Ryder. Things started out OK. Ryder was sitting with us, being good; then without warning, he bolted into the adjacent room in which a private party was being held. Hot on his trail, I found him sitting at a full table of party guests. He saw me approaching and stuck his finger right up his nose; one of his go-to moves. As I got closer, he put that same finger into his mouth; another go-to move when he knows he is being naughty. Amid the stares of the aghast dining guests, I managed to bring Ryder back to our table. I soon regained my own composure, thinking that Ryder had finished bolting and was ready to eat his dinner. BAM! Off again! This time he ran toward the front of the restaurant, which faces a busy street. Thankfully, he hooked a right into another dining area of the restaurant and not a left out into the street. I saw him take a seat at a booth for two with an older couple. Ryder linked his arm under the lady's forearm as I prayed, *Lord Jesus, please don't let him touch their food.*

I approached slowly and calmly and said, "Ryder, you have to come with Mommy." To his emphatic, "No!" I said, "Ryder, come on now, you have to come with Mommy." The lady smiled at me and said, "Oh, he can stay here. He's so cute."

This is very true. Ryder *is* cute, with his rounded bowl haircut, and big, beaming smile he can appear positively angelic. Also, Ryder can be very touchy and loving; so, at that moment, I understood how this might be a beautiful little moment for this woman to share with a surrogate grandson. She didn't know that the scene could go bad without warning and that she could wind up with Ryder screaming and hanging onto her with and iron-clad grip as I try to wrestle him out of the small booth. Thankfully, after the third repetition of, "*You have to come with Mommy*" and the promise of ice cream, Ryder got up calmly, took my hand, and walked away with me. Our ABA training is working.

My understanding of ABA therapy in two words—ABA for Dummies—is: "First…Then." *First* you do this for me, *then* you earn a reward.

I cannot end the chapter without mentioning the controversy that surrounds ABA. Many adult autistics have claimed that it was traumatic for them growing up. They feel that rather than being told to embrace what makes them different, ABA, as a methodology, forced them to conform to be more like typical people. I've heard the methodology compared to child abuse and the conversion therapy that some in the LGBTQ community have been forced to endure. Obviously, to think that Ryder might one day feel this or think that I am at odds on this one subject with some in a community of people I very much love is extremely upsetting. In an effort to learn more about their position, I've asked them what they would consider a suitable alternative treatment for some of Ry's struggles and they have responded, "Try to reason with him or explain the hazards of some of his behavior" or "love him through these things." Unfortunately, I don't have the benefit of being able to do this. We're not talking about a little hand flapping here. I don't care if typical people look at Ry and think he's odd. I love that he's odd. Ryder's tendencies are dangerous and sometimes shocking, we can't afford to wait and see if he slowly grows out of them; and as for appealing to his reason, he is not yet cognitive enough to debate this. Someday, if he's upset that we chose this path, we will deal with it as a family; upset or happy, I guarantee I will be ecstatic that he could even express himself at all because, currently, he is unable to—and I will wonder what role ABA had in the process.

In the meantime, as for "loving" him through it, I love him through everything—every single breath—however misguided some of our decisions may turn out to have been. It's pretty much no different from any decisions made in typical parenting.

16

ANATOMY OF **an Elopement**

I've described eloping incidents and the anxiety they have caused. Since eloping and bolting are such stressful behaviors, I've done plenty of reading and researching in an effort to understand, and hopefully, resolve them. I have reduced the phenomena to several key factors.

The first phase of a successful elopement includes *distraction*, which leads to *opportunity*. The two elements work in tandem. For example, the afternoon that my dad was "watching" the boys. The landscapers had worked earlier in the day while the boys were at school so the yard was manicured and inviting; the boys and my dad were sitting outside. TJ asked my dad a question. In the split second that my dad, distracted, turned his head to answer TJ, Ryder seized the opportunity to run through the gate inadvertently left open by the gardeners. The open gate was an irresistible invitation to Ryder, who doesn't know he's doing anything wrong. For Ryder, that opening may as well have had a flashing neon sign saying, *Walk through here and out. It'll be fun!*

Next comes *doubt* and *uncertainty*. During this phase, precious time can be lost. The caretaker often thinks, *Nah! He couldn't have gotten out; he has to be here someplace.* In fact, you just saw him so he has to be close. Once my dad saw the open gate, he should have known that Ryder was out, instead, he assumed he wasn't and checked the house first. This is a tough but critical moment. You have to check *somewhere* first, and the house or a secure area seems the most logical place to start the search. Instinctually, a typical kid does have some understanding that he or she shouldn't leave the property. A kid with autism and a penchant for eloping lacks this sensibility. There was a case of a high school-aged autism boy who got out of his school; people who passed him on the street didn't even think twice about it. After all, older kids are often on their own; seeing one alone outside is not especially noteworthy. But this boy was not a typical kid, even though his appearance was ordinary. It took some time before the school realized he was missing that day. Tragically, he ran into trouble and weeks later was found dead.

In Ryder's case, because he was so young, his appearance, outside and alone, should have raised a huge red flag for anyone who saw him. Nevertheless, while my dad believed Ryder was in or near the house, Ryder had more time to wander.

The next phase of elopement continues to *realization* and *reaction*. The time it takes to figure out what to do, provides more time for the ASD child to encounter danger. In our case, my dad also had TJ, who was only 7 at the time, under his care. He couldn't split the search with him and go in different directions. With TJ in hand, my dad quickly checked the house and the property around the house. It became clear that Ryder had indeed eloped and the clock was ticking. Dad had to go in search of Ryder; more decisions had to be made. Did Ryder turn left out of the gate or did he turn right? Did he stick to a route that was familiar or did he go off on a new adventure? My dad chose to take a direction that Ryder had taken before and one that led to a favorite destination—the park.

Finally, we come to the *recovery, result,* and *regrouping* phase. There are two ways elopement incidents end: happily or sadly. Luckily, Ryder was small enough to raise concern of some passersby. Ryder was safely recovered, and it was time to regroup.

A safe recovery offers the gift of a second chance and an immediate start at safeguarding. No system is 100 percent effective, but there are a number of steps that can be taken to protect your child. Your child's IEP should clearly state that eloping is an issue and that diligent watch needs to be maintained by school personnel. As I mentioned earlier, alerting neighbors and providing them with your contact information is essential. At home, locks and alarms on doors and windows provide physical protection for your son or daughter and some mental protection for you. Finally, a tracking device on your child is a remarkable use of some of our GPS technology.

Elopement can be considered in definable phases. First, distraction and opportunity working together to incite the getaway. Next, there is doubt and uncertainty that provide critical time for the eloper to follow his or her imagination into freedom. The third phase is the realization of the problem and the reaction to it; deciding what to do first can again put distance between the caregivers and the child. Finally, there is recovery, result, and regrouping. A successful recovery allows parents and caregivers the opportunity to put additional safeguards in place.

Are you ready for your test?

17

Acceptance

I have accepted that Ryder has autism.

You have followed my journey from denial to resistance to doubt, and we have arrived at acceptance. I have accepted that there is no definitive cure, only that higher levels of functioning can be achieved. I have accepted that God, in his infinite wisdom, gave me a child with autism. I am thankful that I am married to a man who is on the same page; one who thinks there is nothing more important than helping our son achieve his full potential. I am thankful that I am married to a man who has willingly taken on a second job to cover the expenses of the additional services that Ryder needs to reach that potential. I am thankful that I am blessed with parents who have sacrificed a great deal to help me and Steve and to love both our boys.

Acceptance of my circumstances and sincere gratitude for my blessings do not negate my sadness. I often feel sad for TJ, who does not have a typical brother. I'm sad for Steve, who is not able to share as much of himself with Ryder as he can with TJ. Ryder is never going to plop down on the couch next to Steve on a Sunday and say, "What's the Jets' score, Dad?" There are two boys—brothers—close in age, who live around the corner. One day, I drove past their house on my way home from work and saw a basketball hoop that had been hung over the garage. I didn't see the boys, just the hoop. I imagined the brothers going outside after school or dinner and shooting baskets together, easily and naturally. I had to pull over and have a quiet moment before I continued home.

One Saturday afternoon, I invited two of TJ's friends to join me and TJ for pizza and to go and see the movie, *Antman*. Both boys were available and happy to have a fun play date. The moms dropped the boys off at the house. All the boys, even Ryder, ran around the house having fun before we headed out. When it was time to go, I said, "Come on guys, we have to leave now." TJ, Brandon, and Christopher eagerly grabbed their jackets and started to the door; Ry followed. Steve jumped up and said, "No, Ry, you stay home with Daddy." I had to swallow the lump in my throat before I continued out with the boys. Steve saw it on my face and mouthed, "It's OK."

We went for pizza, saw the movie. I listened to the three boys rattle on about all the nonsensical things boys talk about. A few times I thought, *My other child, only 21 months younger than his brother, should be here.* The movie was entertaining, the pizza was delicious, and the boys had a great time. They thanked me and waved to TJ when I dropped them off at their houses on our way home.

Back home, I found Ryder asleep on my bed. I lifted him into my arms and cradled him and said through tears, "You'll be able to come to the movies someday. I love you bud." Then TJ approached the bed and gently kissed his brother. "I can't wait until you can come to the movies with me and my friends, Ry," he whispered.

Acceptance   71

That night, TJ's words gave me exactly what I needed to smile and move forward. There have been countless times like this one—times when contrast pulls me up short and tightens my throat. I have come far with my acceptance of autism and the ways it has challenged life as we imagined it would be.

Acceptance was one step in my autism journey.

—⁄⁄⁄—

Having finally accepted Ryder's autism did not mean that I was ready to share it with the outside world. That took time. Eventually, though, I began to go public, slowly, with a hint on Facebook; an autism meme or two shared. And then, after months of dipping my toes into the water, I dove in. I shared posts about Ryder having autism as if I had always been open and public about it. Ryder was becoming older and his delays were becoming more noticeable. No one needed to whisper about my kid behind my back or speculate about what was wrong. I was me again: an open book, willing to face the world head-on.

I threw myself into Autism Awareness Day that year. Ryder and I dressed in blue; I took time off from work and went to his school to frost cookies with blue icing. With the other autism classroom moms, I took pictures to post on the school website and my private page: "We celebrate Autism Awareness Day."

I imagined that every other autism parent would applaud the postings of the children and my participation in the day. Not so. I recall the time when a family member posted an open letter by an autism mom of three daughters, all of whom are on the spectrum, that went viral. Her letter about the varying severity of their autism was heartbreaking. This mom viewed the celebration held on Autism

Awareness Day as a contradiction: there was nothing to celebrate; plenty to criticize. Her letter, and it was not the only one, forced me to think about my actions—and the blue wreath hanging on my front door beneath the blue porch light. Was it wrong to celebrate Autism Awareness Day? I sat and thought about it. I really, really thought about it. When it came down to it, I respected that mother and her feelings as much as I've ever respected anyone; I respected the moms and dads who felt angry and on many levels, and I agreed with them. For me, however, *awareness* means focus; focus means money; money means research; research means support and services. Awareness can come in the form of a protest or a party with cookies iced in blue. I have chosen to advocate, and sometimes, to advocate through celebration. The approach might not be for everyone, but the result will be worthwhile as awareness is heightened and progress is made in understanding the complexities of autism.

Since that first Autism Awareness Day, I have encountered different perspectives and given the issue more thought. I continued to encounter anger on the issue, especially after I wrote, "I don't know why people say children *suffer* from autism, I think my son quite enjoys his." That is, after exhaustion, relief and then laughter following one of Ryder's exploits. One parent responded, "I beg to differ with you. My son does indeed suffer from it. His brother suffers from it. It is a disease, not a disability. Autism sucks." I responded then, and continue to write now, about how proud I am of both of my kids: my autistic son, because of how he deals with the struggles and, how my typical son deals with it all. I have often thought about the parent who called autism a disease. I had never thought in detail whether it was a disorder, a disability, or a disease. But maybe that's just it: it's a broad spectrum.

18

AUTISM AWARENESS
Could Use Some Awareness

We're living in an age during which awareness of differences is emphasized and *acceptance* is the buzz word for the culturally and politically correct among us. This is good. I've learned, however, that all that glitters is not gold and awareness and acceptance aren't always as they seem.

For example, consider Ryder, who, at this point, is "incapable" of following rules, to a local "jumpy place." This play arena has trampolines, each inside a six by eight feet square space, framed by cushioned beams which serve as partitions and protection. Each square is an inner part of a larger section of trampoline cubicles. Children use the beams to move from one square to another, as long as the destination is an empty square; otherwise, they are not allowed to spend any length of time on the beams.

Most of the parents, including Steve, stand on the sidelines half-watching their kids jump and bounce and rebound. Not me. I get right in there, jumping with Ryder. There was a time when I would have felt uncomfortable as the oldest jumper in the arena; now, I do what I have to do to monitor Ryder. Sometimes it works.

Ryder and I were jumping in the biggest of the trampoline sections, comprised of about sixty individual "jumpy squares." The other children in this area were jumping nicely, each on his or her assigned square, following the rules. Sometimes a kid would exit his square to go to another empty square, balancing on the cushioned frame for a short period of time, only as a means to move to a different unoccupied jumpy square. Everything was going well until Ryder began to run wildly from one occupied square to the next occupied square utilizing the frames for balance and speed, catapulting at least two young girls off their trampolines in his wake. I tried to reach him to tell him to stop. I, too, used the cushioned beams and the square trampolines for hurtling across distances; I was certainly not moving as fast as a nimble child. Ryder saw me coming and picked up his getaway speed. I was closing in until an over-sized, 14-year-old boy bounced into my square with enough force to enable him to literally *fly* into the next square. The force made me fall flat. I struggled to straighten up and regain my balance while keeping my eye on Ryder. There was nothing to lean on to pull myself up.

I crawled back onto the beam, almost all the way back, in fact, when a second kid bounced in and, *BAM*, I was down again, this time landing on my back. I looked just like a turtle lying upside down on its shell trying helplessly to right itself. I was still trying to keep my eye on Ryder; there was danger that he would get out, not only of the section, but of the building itself. Luckily, I saw him, running from beam to beam, leaving dazed kids in a tumble behind him.

And I saw Steve, standing safely on solid ground looking at me in disbelief and horror. Like I wanted to be in this predicament?

I called out to him and signaled for help. He shook his head *no*. *No?* How could this be a reasonable response?

Finally, TJ bounced over and helped me up. I tried to regain my composure as we made it to the group of other parents chatting with Steve. I stood on the sidelines and watched Ryder breaking all the rules. I listened to TJ and Steve reenacting my whole embarrassing experience; they were having a grand old time laughing it up: "No, she looked more like this…"

And then I felt the stares of the other parents as the red-shirted manager approached with righteous purpose. I am no longer phased by the stares of onlookers, and I am no longer surprised when Steve tries to distance himself from any upcoming embarrassment. It's his way of coping. I am surprised by anyone who stands in judgment.

The manager began, "Ma'am, your son is not following the rules…" As I was listening to the reprimand, I saw Ryder off in the distance with a big happy smile on his face, running—and *Ooops*—there went another catapulted jumper.

"I know, Sir," I answered with mustered sincerity, "I'm sorry. My son doesn't follow rules because he doesn't understand them. He has autism."

"Ma'am, we're worried about his safety."

"Don't worry, he'll be fine. I'd be happy to sign a waiver so that you are not responsible for his safety. Would that do it?" I offered this calmly and politely, suppressing my frustration and anger; I knew the manager did not want to understand or accept. He wanted me and Ryder out. I offered to take Ryder to a different jumpy section, away from the other kids. Even the manager's awareness of my son's issue did not allow him to compromise.

"I actually don't have one that will work for him right now," he said after a quick scan of the arena. "I can give you free passes to come back another day. We have special jump times for children like yours."

What I've found is that often, the "special" times are the "off" times, the times, for example, when the venue is not in use by other kids who have evening homework to do. The awareness of children with autism is not always inclusive and is often intolerant, popular news feeds notwithstanding. Perhaps this manager could have worked with me to find an acceptable compromise: maybe a supervised time-out for Ryder and a return to a more isolated trampoline area. More broadly, perhaps the "special" times could be within the popular weekend times, like the adult swim times at community pools. Perhaps *awareness* needs to be strengthened with sensitivity and genuine acceptance.

That day, I relented. "OK we'll go," I said, "but you have to get him for me. I tried catching him and I couldn't." The manager quickly agreed, having absolutely no idea of what catching Ryder might entail.

As the manager left to collect Ryder I noticed TJ was tearing up, disappointed we had to leave. I said to him, "Go ahead, Babe, go back to the squares and jump for a bit longer. This is going to take a while."

And it did!

19

STEPHEN'S Turn

Steve has a law enforcement background. He served two years with the New York Police Department. He was an officer in uniform in the Courts for over ten years before passing the test to become a Supreme Court clerk. Steve definitely has a follow-the-rules personality. He checks and rechecks things not only at work, but at home as well; he makes sure the oven is off and the appliances are unplugged several times before leaving the house. We have a pool in our backyard that at its deepest is ten feet. The pool is surrounded by a gated, mesh fence. Steve ensures that the gate is locked when either of us are not swimming with the boys. Steve knows the protocols for watching Ryder and uses his no-nonsense, extra-careful skill set when he is in charge. Usually.

One Friday evening, Steve had to attend an event at Belmont Racetrack. He asked me to leave work on time so that he could leave with his friend, Charlie, who was due to pick him up at the same time I usually get home from work. I was just about to turn off the big boulevard that leads to my house when my phone rang: Steve was trying to reach me. I answered and without even the perfunctory *hello*, I said, "Calm down; I'm almost home."

"No, wait…he's OK."

After the reassurance, Steve continued, "Ryder got over the pool fence. Deb, it happened in just a second."

"I'll be right home."

I sped into the driveway, leaving tire skids on the road. Steve answered the door, soaking wet. His clothes, even his shoes were leaving puddles on the floor. I followed him into the backyard and saw that a whole panel of the pool fence had been ripped out of the ground. It must've been like a scene from *The Incredible Hulk*. Steve said that the pool gate key jammed in the lock when he tried to open the gate and run to Ryder, who looked as if he was struggling in the water. More likely, the gate didn't open right away and Steve, panicked, tore it, and the connected fence, out of the ground. Ryder had been taking autism swim lessons at the Y, and I had him practice swimming to the ladder at home; nevertheless, neither Steve nor I ever left Ryder alone in the pool.

Steve said that Ryder had been playing in a different section of the yard with his toys, so he quickly ran to get chlorine tablets from the shed nearby. When he came out, he saw the last of Ry's feet going over the pool fence. Steve yelled, "Ryder, stay there!" Ryder looked back at him and jumped right into the deep end of the pool.

Believe me, I knew exactly how he felt. The gate was wrecked, but Steve and Ryder were OK.

No matter how often Ryder eloped, he never did so to be naughty or defiant. From his perspective, he ran when he saw opportunity for some fun or exploration. Opportunity, for Ryder, was an invitation.

When my locksmith cousin came to install new locks, we asked him to secure the doors and not to worry about the windows. We had never ever seen Ryder show any interest in the windows. In fact, he usually avoided them: noisy things like mowers and leaf blowers were out there. If Ryder needed to look out of the window for something, he would creep up to where his eyes were just above the sill to peek out.

One Sunday afternoon, Steve stayed home with Ryder while I took TJ to his flag football game. When we got home, TJ got out of the car and ran into the house; I stayed in the car in the driveway to send a quick text to a girlfriend. When I got out of the car, I looked up and saw Ryder standing on the outside sill of his open bedroom window. He was on the second story of the house: one arm holding the inside wall of his room; the other holding the outside wall of the house. He was looking down.

I raced to stand directly below him. I screamed for Steve as loudly as I could. I couldn't run inside to find Steve for fear that Ryder would jump or fall, and I wouldn't be there to catch him. I couldn't call Steve on my cell phone because I'd have to take my eyes off Ry. I couldn't even extend my arms because we do that sometimes while Ryder's on his bed or the couch to invite him to jump into our arms. I didn't want Ryder to think I was inviting him to jump! I stood frozen in place, braced to try to break his fall. I was, of course, imagining the worse.

Then I saw Steve's arm wrap around Ryder's waist and pull him back inside, back to the toys that they had been playing with just moments before.

My extra-careful Steve had left Ryder for one minute to run to the bathroom.

Needless to say, locks and alarms are now on the windows.

20

WRECK IT, **Ryder**

Every so often, Ryder tosses his room, completely upending it. When it happens once, it kicks off a series of "tossings," sometimes up to sixteen in a row. He strips the bed of blankets, pillows, and any stuffed animals or toys. On the really bad nights, he removes the mattress, too—yes, he finds the strength to hurl the mattress off the top bunk!

While his room seems mostly secured, Ryder inevitably manages to find something that evaded both Steve's and my radar. One night, Ryder came into in my room chewing on something white. I quickly made him open up so I could scoop out whatever was in his mouth. I excavated a few pieces of what looked like the white Styrofoam "snow" that often comes as packaging. My antennae shot up: this was a signal that trouble was afoot. I went into Ryder's room to find the source of his "snack." When I opened the door, I saw a virtual winter wonderland that had overtaken his room. I looked until I found the source of the fluff blanketing the room: one of TJ's two Ninja Turtle bean bags. One of them had the misfortune of having a loose string hanging from its stitching. When Ryder spied the inviting thread, he pulled and pulled until a hole developed. Then he wriggled two fingers inside, pulled the opening wider, and relieved the bean bag of all the stuffing. While Steve cursed and vacuumed, Ryder, his hands over his ears to muffle the noise, jumped onto my lap to be quieted and comforted.

Steve opposed my approach; he has a more traditional view of the consequences that should follow wayward behaviors. It's during times like these when I wonder whether there is any definitive right or wrong answer to the question of the best way to handle things with Ryder.

I described how Ryder tossed his room to our ABA team leader, Karrie. Karrie's first suggestion was to let him toss the bedroom, and then make him help us clean it up. We should try, she said, to make cleanup part of the tossing ritual.

Getting Ryder to help clean up after a tossing was a major failure.

The next thing Karrie theorized was that this could be a good thing, developmentally. Ryder was never particularly aware of specific things as a toddler. This tossing behavior, she speculated, reflected Ryder testing his capabilities and his boundaries. He hadn't done the mischievous things kids do during toddlerhood; now, more aware, he was doing them. Although the thought that I was to experience the terrible twos with Ryder four years after the fact did not evoke that *hip-hip hooray* moment for me, I was happy to consider the wrecking behavior as a breakthrough.

Karrie may be on to something, though. My parents have a dog, Lucy, since before Ryder was born. Ryder lived in the same house with the dog for years. In all that time, I never saw Ryder interact with the dog. I didn't even notice that I had never seen him interact with the dog until the first night that he did. We were sitting in the living room after dinner, chatting. Ryder walked past us, with Lucy on her leash. Ryder was saying, "Walk, please walk. Walk, please walk," in a gravelly, robotic-like voice. It's how he talks. (Hopefully, when he really masters language and gets more confident, he'll sound more natural. Right now, though, he does sound like, God help me, Regan, the possessed child in *The Exorcist*.) Anyway, as he was walking Lucy around the living room, Steve turned to me and said, "Well, look who realized we have a dog." Once Steve said this out loud, we realized that Ryder seriously either didn't know or didn't care that we had a dog, and then he did. I chose to interpret it as the progress that Karrie was describing.

I have another theory, which has to do with one of Ryder's autism traits. TJ wears colorful yellow and green Incredible Hulk T-shirts and other superhero shirts. When I try to put one on Ryder, he pushes the shirt away and states firmly, "No!" If I somehow get it on him before he realizes which graphic is on the front, once he sees it, he will not stop squirming until he gets it off his body. I'd like to say the child has carefully considered tastes, but this is one of his autism things: the T-shirt has too much going on creating too much sensory overload. It's the same with his bedding: the sheets, the comforters, and the throw pillows have to be solid colors. No explosion of colors and superhero graphics. Like the removal of the tee off his body, so went the original, wildly colorful bedding off his bed.

Ryder's doing a little better with tossing the room these days. I still don't make him clean up afterward, though. I know I should take Karrie's expert advice, but I've become accustomed to ending my night by cleaning up the room after a tossing event as Ryder sleeps. It serves as the reminder that although all sorts of chaotic crap could've gone on during the day, in the end, I will regain control and put everything back together for as long as Ryder needs me to do that—and for as long as I need me to do that.

21

MY MARRIAGE **and Autism**

I do not hold to the belief that there is that one true soul-mate for each of us. It sounds beautiful in theory, but I happen to think the most important factors in finding a mate are luck and timing. I was lucky to meet Steve when I did and luckier still to marry him. But this is not a mushy-gushy warm and fuzzy love story. It's about the reality of living with someone every day, paying bills, doing household chores, being spread thinly with children's activities, and harboring resentments from wrongdoing's over the course of a relationship's lifetime. These factors are what makes up a marriage and, if not kept in check, they can chip away at it. The fire of the initial romance we have at age 25 mellows over time!

I remember during our Pre-Cana class, the speaker declared, "You should love no one above your spouse, except for God." I had an inkling even then, before Steve and I had children, that there would be no way that I would love anyone above my own children. And now with them here, I realize I love them way more than I imagined I would before they came along.

Steve was a friend long before he became a lover. Our parents were friendly. We knew each other for years and even tried dating once or twice before romance finally stuck. Before that, I was attracted to the bad-boy types, while Steve spent a lot of time dating casually, not seeming to care if he ever found anyone special.

When you really come down to it, the idea of marriage is strange: it's a commitment for the rest of your life to someone based on feelings and passions that you are having at a young age. You bring to this union the limited experiences and practices from the life you've led thus far, and most likely different from the backstory the other person is bringing to the union. You must intertwine these two differing backgrounds and somehow sort through them to make them work together over a shared lifetime. There is compromising when you're able to, standing your ground when you absolutely need to, and giving in to keep the peace when you can stand to cave. And through all this, you need to maintain your feelings and physical attraction to the person.

Here's a story that tells lots about me and Steve and all that I have just said. Steve's dad is a former Marine. He raised his boys to be strong and independent. Like his dad, Steve takes pride in fixing things around the house without calling in—or paying for—outside help. The main toilet in our house was 52 days in to not working…efficiently. It was making a strange noise after it was flushed. So, per Steve, after we flushed, we were supposed to lift the tank top up and pull up and hold a little box for a few seconds. But we couldn't do that immediately after a flush because the little box wasn't ready to be lifted until a few minutes *after* the flush. I begged Steve to call a plumber to fix the toilet once and for all. "Why spend 200 dollars on a plumber," he countered, "just because you won't hold up a little piece of plastic for a few seconds?"

One day we were about to head out to Ryder's special soccer playgroup, which Ryder calls *baskball*. I went to the bathroom then headed out to the car. Steve was inside doing his clean sweep, double-check of the house before we left. The boys and I waited in the car, Ryder repeating, "I go baskball. I play baskball."

A few minutes passed and Steve did not come out of the house. I sent TJ in to ask what the holdup was. TJ returned to the car and said, "Daddy says you didn't flush right again, Mom, and so he has to wait to fix it."

Ryder continued, "I play baskball."

I told TJ to get back inside the car and watch Ryder. I got out of the car, slammed the door, and stormed inside. "Come on Stephen, let's go!"

"We can't, I have to wait for the tank to fill to flush it again the right way."

"There's not supposed to be a right or wrong way to flush an f'ing toilet! It's supposed to be one of the things in life you're not supposed to put any thought into. If we can't just flush and go about our lives, it's time to call a plumber!"

I went back to the car, huffing and puffing, and ready to blow the house down. Steve followed. After a few minutes he said, "We need a new toilet."

"You don't know that; let's get a plumber in. It could be a quick fix, a replacement part that costs fifty dollars. Let's just see, Steve."

With Ry's declaration, "I go baskball!" we were off.

If it had been up to me, I would have followed in my parents' footsteps, and we would've called a plumber in immediately. During our years together, I have to come around to accepting Steve as being frugal, and he has to come around to my rebellious haphazard flushing ways until

I can finally convince him to get the job done by someone who knows what he's doing—*damn-the-cost* way of operating. Somehow, we balance each other.

I've read that 80 percent of marriages that involve raising a child with autism end in divorce. I'd be lying if I said I didn't see how that is probable. As I've explained, we can't take our eyes off Ryder; we can't plop him in front of the TV for an hour or send him over to a friend's house for a night so that we can have time alone for some fun, some sex, some intimacy. We can't have date nights because we can't just get a random babysitter for Ryder. The only competent babysitters for our child have to be the people who have an understanding of the dangerous level of his capabilities. The only way to gain this understanding is to see Ryder day in and day out. My babysitters are my parents. My parents do after-school babysitting duty every day of the school week. My mom and dad are elderly; I can't ask them to do weekends, too. It would be unfair.

Want to laugh? The last time Steve and I had hot, spontaneous sex was on the floor of our hotel bathroom in Mexico, during our ten-year anniversary trip. This, while the boys were half-asleep in the bed fifty feet outside our door. The whole time that I was cavorting on the tile floor, I was wondering if Ryder had missed the bowl while he was peeing earlier that day and if my hair was mopping up his urine. Even when Ryder should not be on my mind, he finds a way to be there, front and center. Sometimes at the most inappropriate times.

Whenever I feel that my marriage is struggling, I recall a favorite memory. One late-July afternoon, Steve and I took our two boys to Wantagh Pool for an outing with my autism support group. I usually don't like to visit crowded places with Ryder, but I thought that if the rest of the parents and kids were going, we could go, too. So off the four of us went.

There was a lot of ground to walk across there, just getting from the parking lot to the entrance, and it was overwhelming. Then there was the long line of people waiting to sign up and pay to get inside the complex. When we finally got in, the pool and surrounding playground area was crowded and chaotic. Ryder, of course, found the spot he enjoyed best: a water park section with slides and ladders and lots of sprinklers throughout. TJ agreed to hang out there as well, even though it was geared toward much younger children. While TJ was climbing and sliding on his own, Steve and I were watching Ryder. Steve stood on one side of a water structure, I stood on the other side, and Ryder was happily slipping and sliding between us. Steve and I were rather far apart, separated by the wide slide. It didn't take us long, though, to come up with a way to communicate despite the distractions of the kids and the noise and the splashing going on between us: we were hand signaling like a practiced catcher with his pitcher. It was and remains the perfect metaphor for our life together. We work together, come up with a system, and make it work.

Despite the toll that Ryder has taken on us, and therefore our marriage, I am still insanely attracted to Steve. Sometimes, when we're all dressed up going to a wedding or a party, or when Steve gets a little tan from the sun, his handsomeness actually takes my breath away. There is no one I respect more than Steve. There is *nothing* in this world I hold more sacred than our vows and the commitment we made to each other; even if it's tested regularly—and Ryder makes sure it's tested regularly!

22

SIBLING **Love**

There are things autism teaches that couldn't possibly be learned without its insistent presence.

One day, a woman in my autism support group shared a story about the night she went to her neuro-typical son's Open School Night at the beginning of his school year. The second-grade kids were asked to write a note to their parents describing what they'd do with a million dollars. The boys and girls wrote variations of a trip to Disney World, a visit to the real Jurassic Park, and even a "no school" calendar. My fellow autism mom looked down at her son's paper, which had, "find a cure for autism."

Our neuro-typical siblings are not choosing to learn about the tolerance and patience that autism demands, they are, without option, living it. They're not faking their compassion when they express it. They see firsthand all that autism gives and all it takes. The problem is, we, their parents, are learning about it at the same time, so it's not as if we have a store of advice or guidance to give them.

We took on this commitment of parenting for better or for worse, our other children didn't.

Siblings of an autism child usually have not lived too many years, if any, without his or her diagnosed brother or sister. Sometimes, the obvious has to be explained. I remind TJ, "There are things a regular brother does that Ryder doesn't. A regular brother would probably like the same toys as you and would probably play with you. But he might steal your toys from you or hide them to try to fool you! Ryder doesn't do that." The message registers: TJ is quite possessive about his toys. This will be understood more deeply as TJ matures. I tell him that he is learning lessons about patience and compromise that his friends will have to learn later in life. I try to explain to him that no one in this life gets away with not having something they need to deal with or some challenge they must overcome. I think he gets this.

TJ is acutely aware and considerate of the needs of his brother. There are times when we'll be leaving the house, and before the door is opened, TJ will be the one who says, "Who has Ryder?" As a family, we share a Ryder-responsibility inventory: *Do you have Ryder? Will you take Ryder?* Raising the two boys is a balancing act: on the one hand, I don't want TJ to grow to resent Ryder; but on the other hand, I do want him to learn the responsibility that autism demands from each of us.

I try to do special things just for TJ. He made his Holy Communion this year. Steve wanted a quiet luncheon with only family; I wanted a big, over the top, 100-person, catered party, complete with music and decorations and plenty of food. "Steve," I said, "so much is about Ryder. TJ needs a full day when it's all about him." Steve agreed, and we got busy.

We planned a big event. A few days before his special day, TJ told me that he wanted the DJ to announce his entrance to the party to Bruno Mars' "Uptown Funk." I found a pair of small, black-rimmed sunglasses for him to wear. On the big day, wearing the glasses and his First Communion suit, he looked like a smaller, more handsome, John Belushi from the *Blues Brothers*. I took my seat, the music started, and TJ strutted into the room, stepped to dead center of the dance floor, and broke into a full-on choreographed hip-hop dance routine. Steve later confessed that he believed that this was something TJ and I had practiced. We did not. In fact, I was as shocked as the other 98 guests. It was such a moment! I still return to the video to watch our friends and family cheer TJ. TJ needed the celebration; the day was all about him. I had the good sense to hire Ryder's ABA, Rebecca, to stay with him at the party for the day; TJ enjoyed our undivided attention. Before he fell asleep later that night, he said, "Mom, today was the best day ever." It really was.

While TJ can certainly wow a crowd, he is also very quiet, confidant, self-assured. One day he was telling me a story about his class trip to the museum. He also told me about the bus trip back. He said, "No kids sat next to me, mom. But don't worry, Mrs. Decker sat with me." My heart broke for my son. TJ is not drawn to sports in this sports-oriented suburb. I confess that I worry about his social growth. I know, though, that TJ is comfortable in his own skin and has friends when he wants a play date. TJ's teacher has reassured me that he is well-liked by the other kids in his class. I was upset that TJ sat alone on the bus, but TJ seemed OK with it. I know you know me by now: I worry about my kids; both of them.

Autism has given TJ a strong sense of empathy. This has been an unexpected bonus of autism. I can't say this happens in every family with an autism child. One woman in my support group, which has a sibling support component, joined because her typical son, a year younger than her child with autism, was not developing empathy toward his brother. Several times, under different circumstances, he was leading the charge and encouraging other children to make fun of his brother. This is often a defense or coping mechanism, but it still must be heartbreaking for her. I count my blessings. TJ may be embarrassed by his brother as he moves through puberty. Right now, though, he's not. Ryder went through a phase where he panted like a dog; TJ thought it was funny. I imagine something like this won't be amusing when TJ brings his first girlfriend home. I should save my worry about things like this for the future, and keep my mind focused on the here and now. And now, TJ and Ryder get along great, without friction. Ryder leaves for school before TJ does. Each morning when Ryder leaves, TJ is up and at the door to be sure to say goodbye to his little brother. God forbid I should not wake TJ up for their daily, dramatic morning goodbye. Some mornings I have to laugh to myself. I restrain from reminding TJ that Ryder is going to kindergarten, not off to war.

One afternoon, we were going to a birthday party for one of Ryder's classmates, a boy with Down syndrome. I did not know whether or not TJ had ever seen a Down syndrome person before. I didn't know if he'd blurt out something about Jacob's appearance. I stressed throughout the drive to the party wondering, *Should I bring it up beforehand? Do I not say anything? Oh my God, what if he says something in front of Jacob's mother?* I decided to have a talk with TJ.

"TJ," I said, "all these kids here today will be different, like Ryder's different. Let's be patient today, OK? Also, Sweetie, if you have questions about the children, you come and whisper them to mommy. Don't say anything out loud in front of someone else's mommy because maybe the question will hurt the kid's mommy's feelings." I hoped TJ was listening.

The party went well. Cake, ice cream, no drama. On the way back home, TJ told me he thought Jacob was adorable. And he meant it. TJ seeks Jacob out and sticks by him at special soccer games or at the park. Jacob has a typical brother, Joseph, who is TJ's age and has the same interests as TJ; the two older boys have developed a nice friendship with the unique bond of atypical brothers.

As the older brother of an autism sibling, TJ has to contend with some important issues. When the good weather arrived this spring, I had to sit down with TJ and have one of our talks. "TJ," I began, "if your brother runs into the street when you're together, you can't run after him. You can yell. You can try to grab him, but only go as far as the curb; you have to stop at the curb before the street." One day before we had this talk, TJ was so focused on catching Ryder that he ran into the street after his brother. His response to my warning was, "But if I don't try to stop him, he may get hit by a car."

"TJ, if you run into the street, you could *both* get hit by a car. Don't worry, TJ, the ABA girls are going to teach Ryder not to run into the street. You'll see, no one will be running into the street by the end of the summer."

TJ was not buying it. A look of concern came over his face. I don't know how to spare him these worries when I barely know how to quell them within myself, so our talks will continue. Along with our patience and our love.

23

RYDER TAKES *the Stage*

We were invited to a bowling party—TJ was almost 6 and Ryder almost 4. The party was for Christopher, who lives across the street. This was before the bolting and eloping incidents became a common occurrence but after the first Actionland incident. Let's just say that I was somewhat, but not fully, aware of Ryder's capabilities. Somewhere deep down inside, I probably still thought the Actionland thing was exclusive to amusement park rides and climbing.

The bowling party was in August; I wore a light, summery skirt and flip-flops. No sooner did we enter the bowling alley than Ryder broke free from my hand and took off running non-stop down one of the lanes. I took off after him as fast as I could. I couldn't let him reach the end where the pins drop down, the space from which a bowling alley worker might appear to straighten the pins when the automatic pinsetter malfunctions. As I ran after Ryder, God had my back and I somehow managed to stay upright despite the slippery wooden lane and the flip-flopping flip-flops.

"Hey you're not allowed to run down there!" came the voice of a bowling alley authority. With no time to spare, I dove. I had no choice; I was not going to reach my little boy unless I did.

I managed to tackle Ryder onto the lane, the man's admonitions still loud. I got Ryder up. He was laughing. He loved it!

We headed back up the lane to the seating area. I was red-faced and shaking from the near-miss with disaster. The manager approached us and declared, "You're not supposed to run down the lanes; you could have been hurt!"

My voice cracked; barely holding back tears I answered, "Do you really think I *wanted* to run down the lane? Do you think I *wanted* to tackle my child and embarrass myself here?" I was full on crying by then. The man softened and apologized. I was shaking. At that moment, I would have gladly accepted a shot of hard liquor along with his pardon; it was about 11 in the morning.

Every kid with autism has his or her triggers, those things that initiate unpredictable, unnerving behaviors. Among others, one of Ryder's triggers is a stage. I found this out the hard way the first time I took him to a Special Ed PTA dance during his first year of elementary school. After months of believing that his eloping behavior had improved, I walked into the school auditorium holding Ryder's hand. Before I had the chance to settle at our table, Ryder took off toward the stage. He ran up the stage steps, raced behind the DJ, and bolted out an emergency exit behind stage left. He was gone. It was pitch dark backstage. I honestly didn't know which way to give chase. Luckily, the DJ appeared from behind the darkness holding Ryder by the arm.

After a bit, I was able to bribe Ryder to sit at the table with me, offering chicken nuggets and fries. He was sitting nicely for a few minutes when I noticed that look in his eyes. *BAM!* He was off again.

When Ryder knows I'm a just a few steps behind him, he runs wildly to get away from me *unless* he sees something that attracts his attention away from me. That night, as Ryder bolted from our table, he came to a standstill. I panicked and looked around to figure out what had caught his interest and, therefore, in which direction he was likely to charge. Unfortunately, I didn't notice the distraction in time. I was too late. It was a nicely dressed lady walking toward us using a cane for support.

Ryder rushed to her and grabbed the bottom end of the cane. The poor woman held on tightly and thus began a tug of war. Thank goodness that her husband was there to steady her, while I was able to grab Ryder and loosen his grip from her walking stick. So there we were at a special needs event and my special needs son was physically bullying a disabled woman. For her, he was a menace; for him, she was grist in the game mill.

My saving grace was that the room, which doubles as a cafeteria, had a vending machine, another one of Ry's favorite attractions. He attempts to get his hand, arm, or even a whole shoulder through the retrieval bin, not unlike Woody and Buzz do with the toy machine in *Toy Story*. I took Ryder to the vending machine and let him try to climb in; one way or another, I had to get his focus off the stage and away from the woman's cane. Thankfully, no one approached with unsolicited advice about the foolishness of allowing my son to try to climb into the vending machine. At least, I was able to monitor him there. I can't say the same for a disappearance into the back of a darkened stage or a dash for an unsuspecting woman with a cane.

A few weeks after realizing Ryder had a thing for stages, I received a video text from my friend, Kristi, who is on the PTA at his school. The attached text stated, "So this just happened." The clip was of Ryder and his teacher "dancing" on stage. When I called to ask her what exactly I was watching, Kristy explained that the school held an anti-bullying assembly; the DJ asked if anyone wanted to come up and dance on stage. Ryder jumped out of his seat and ran up with his teacher. I played the video back and, of course, I got it. It wasn't this delightful scene in which a little boy chose to dance with his teacher on stage; it was a determined teacher dancing and moving her student around as he incessantly tried to break free and get past her to run to the back of the stage. When Ryder moved to the right, she stopped him and spun him around, encouraging him to shake his hips a little. Then he attempted to get around her on the left; but, nope, she pulled off another forcible turn-around and hip shake. What I was watching was Ryder's repeated effort to bolt, thwarted over and over again by a practiced teacher. It was comical for me to watch, because I knew what his devious mind was thinking. Yet, for everyone in that audience, it was a heartwarming moment of a young autistic boy dancing with his teacher at an anti-bullying assembly.

Recently, the local children's museum hosted an Autism Awareness Day, which included a performance of the play, *Little Red Riding Hood*. It was a free, closed, special event just for autistic children and their families. It included access to the rest of the museum. I signed up for both the play and the museum access. I thought it would be the perfect opportunity to once again test Ryder's ability to sit still in a theatre and watch a play, especially since the audience was going to be that of people who had an understanding of autism.

Steve was working, so my parents offered to accompany me and the boys. They know I like to have at least one other adult with us to watch TJ in case I need to deal with a surprise from Ryder. Immediately before the show, while we were standing in line to go inside the theater, I ran to use the ladies room. I left Ryder with my parents; TJ had gone off with my friend, Linda, and her boys to see an exhibit before the start of the play. As luck would have it, the theatre doors were opened before I returned.

When I finally got inside, I saw my parents seated in the third row with Ryder, but there were no adjacent seats. I ended up joining TJ and Linda in the row behind them, but at the opposite end of the row. In retrospect, I probably should have asked one of my parents to move so that I could take the seat next to Ryder. The play was a two-person play that alternated between hand puppets and two girls who narrated and acted. About five minutes into the performance, Ryder shouted out, "*MILK!*" This was followed by my mom's audible, "*Shhh.*" A few seconds later, there was another shout of "*MILK!*" from Ryder. And then another, "*MILK, PLEASE?!*"

TJ was staring at me with that uncomfortable expression that pleads, *Mom, do something.* Because we were in a room full of understanding and accepting autism families, I decided to give it a little more time and held my breath. Another shout-out, "*Can I have MILK, PLEASE?*"

I had to act; audience focus had turned away from the stage to Ryder. With whispered *excuse mes*, I shimmied myself out of my seat, over the laps and feet of fellow playgoers, and down the row, desperately focused on salvaging the afternoon.

In my haste and concentration to get to Ryder, I didn't notice that the girls performing had moved to a bunk bed in the back of the stage. Bunk beds are another one of Ry's things: he likes structures. Without warning, Ryder switched from his desperate cries for milk to "*I want sleep now!*" And then he was off and running toward the stage and the bed. My Dad did his best to grab him as he leapt into the aisle, but Ryder left his 72-year-old grandfather grabbing at thin air.

I was free of my row and off after him. When I finally caught up to him, Ryder was lifting himself onto the stage, and although his upper body had cleared the edge, I managed a wrestler's grip on his legs. It was a scene, one that rivaled whatever was happening on the stage itself. Ryder and I engaged in a memorable struggle: me, holding for dear life onto his legs while trying to pull him down from the lip of the stage; Ryder, writhing and kicking, determined to get into that bed and go to sleep. Although the action off-stage continued—and even escalated at one point—I did manage to get Ryder quieted and out of the theater with the promise of milk, of course. The actresses continued to perform as if nothing else was going on around them. Those girls are true professionals!

When I recapped the day for Steve, he said, with insight, "I'll bet the girl playing the part of little red riding hood was wishing that the big bad wolf would come on stage and swallow them whole!"

24

KEEPING A *Sense of Humor*

My sense of humor, which I inherited from my father, has always made awkward moments easier, dull moments more fun, and work days go faster. My sense of humor is broad, ranging from sarcastic to slapstick, highbrow to hyperbolic. A strong sense of humor and a love of laughter have served me well. When I was younger, I had an uproarious belly laugh, which quieted for a while over the years but has now returned. I'm laughing again—a lot! The antics of my boys provide the source of much of my happiness. Ryder, naturally, never ceases to spark laughter.

There was an episode of *Seinfeld* in which Jerry's dentist converts to Judaism and immediately starts making Jewish jokes. Jerry, appalled, meets with a Catholic priest to complain about this. The priest asks, "This offends you as a Jewish person?" No, Jerry answers, "It offends me as a comedian." Jerry didn't mind the idea of poking fun at Jews, he minded that the jokes were just not *funny*. In our supposedly politically correct, culturally sensitive world, one would never think to make fun of or accept without protest a joke said at the expense of a person with special needs. Not in our house! Here, it's survival of the fittest, autism notwithstanding. In this family, each of us must be prepared to be the butt of a joke and be willing to laugh at missteps and mishaps.

One of the funniest moments occurred one day when I ran out to meet Ryder at the bus. His matron at the time, Lisa, could be kind of intense and serious. "Oh Deb," she would report, "he tried to get up out of his seat today. If he gets up again, I will have to notify the school and they'll need to restrain him. Remember, one more time, Deb." She reported each of Ryder's movements with assertive sobriety. While I listened to her drone on, I couldn't help but think, *Go for it, Lisa, you show his little ass who is boss!* And then, as the bus pulled away, I had a good laugh.

Another day, when the bus pulled up, Lisa disembarked with Ryder in tow and said, "Oh Deb, we had a problem on the bus today. While we were complimenting another child on his new shoes, Ryder yanked them off his feet." While Lisa frowned, Ryder was happily untying my sneaker laces.

I tried to give Lisa my polite attention, but *really*? The bottom line is that Ryder needs instant feedback: reprimands at the moment of naughty; compliments and praise at the moment of nice. So, although I knew it was too late for a reprimand to have any meaning for Ryder, I made a reasonable show of scolding him when he stepped off the bus. Of course, Ry had no idea what the heck I was talking about. Lisa seemed satisfied.

Later that evening I saw my friend, Linda, at our special soccer group. Remember? Linda's son, Jacob, has Down syndrome; he is in Ryder's class. When I told her the story she said, "They didn't tell me about it when they dropped Jacob off. It had to be Jacob that Lisa was talking about.

He wore his new orthopedic shoes to school today for the first time, and I asked the staff to make a big deal over them because he doesn't like wearing them."

I burst out laughing! First of all, Jacob and Ryder are friends; Ryder *likes* Jacob. Also, Jacob is much smaller than Ryder. Finally, Jacob usually falls asleep on the bus on the short ride home. So I have the picture: Ryder, twice the size of the sleeping Jacob, seizes the orthopedic shoes off his Down syndrome buddy because he likes them, or wants them, or is playing a new game. Lisa bears witness to Ryder's assault on Jacob's feet and wants justice. Maybe she believes this will propel Ryder into a life of crime. Once again, Ryder's antics provided lots of laughs—this time for both me and Linda.

Ryder refers to himself as *Wyder O*. Why? There's a Ryder M. in his class, so this is perfectly reasonable. That's how it's always been when there are a few children in the class with the same first name; they are distinguished by adding the first initial of their last name.

Ryder doesn't realize that once he is outside of the classroom and out of Ryder M.'s presence, he can be just *Ryder*. When I say, "You come here. Who's mommy's baby?" Ryder answers, "Wyder O." I usually say, "Yes, Ryder M's mommy can rest easy tonight; you're my baby. Ryder M. is not."

Whenever anyone asks Ryder his name, he replies, *Wyder O*. The comedians I live with run with this. I came into the living room the other day, and I saw the usual mess of books and toys thrown across the rug and under the furniture. "Who made this mess?" I ask, hands on hips. Steve answers, "Maybe it was *Wyder O*?"

Ryder is no slave to fashion. Often, when we're in a hurry, Steve or I will throw the nearest hat or the most accessible jacket on Ryder, who is always happier about going out than concerned about his haberdashery. One morning, Steve was going to dash out to get some bagels for our breakfast. We were all running late that day; TJ had to get to his religion class, I had to get to work, and Ry had to get dressed and ready for his day. Ryder wanted to go with Steve. With no time for reasoning or for a scene, I looked at Steve and said, "Just take him!"

Ryder had on his red pajamas—short sleeves, short bottoms. Steve grabbed the nearest coat—a dull, green Army jacket. I tossed the hat closest to my hand over to Steve—a blue woolen beanie with a bright yellow pompom. Steve pulled it over Ryder's uncombed hair as I pushed his sockless feet into his sneakers. With six inches of calf exposed between the bottom of his pajamas and the top of his sneakers and the yellow pompom bouncing on top of his head, Ryder grabbed Steve's hand and off they went. TJ waved from the front door. Then he turned to me and said, "Jeez, mom, you let your son go out in public like that?" And then we both laughed, knowing full well that Ryder could not have cared less.

Ryder has two reactions to a scolding: he either covers his ears to block out the noise or he repeats, word-for-word what has been said, only much, much louder. And then he laughs at the game he is playing. It's like he momentarily forgets he doesn't really talk and he spontaneously does. One day, I was driving on the Meadowbrook Parkway with the boys strapped in their car seats in the back. Suddenly, Ryder leaned over the middle console, his face next to mine. He was out of his car seat! I screamed, "Ryder, *sit down!*"

Ryder yelled right back, "Wyder, *shit down!*" and then immediately sat back down and strapped himself in as well. Things quieted down, my heartbeat returned to normal, and, seconds later, 5-year-old TJ said, "Mommy, Ryder said *shit.*" He fully expected me to parent. Really?

I believe that most things in life are made infinitely better when humor is kept in the mix. The goal is to accrue more checks in the "laugh" column than in the "cry" column. Albeit somewhat counterintuitive, autism has greatly improved my sense of humor and given me an outstanding ability to weigh the relative importance of the things that happen each day. Autism has also given me some of my best material, my *schtick*, which I hope you are enjoying.

Ba dump bump! (Mic drop)

25

I PRAYED, *God Laughed*

My relationship with God has evolved. I feel close to him and have attended church throughout my life, albeit with varying degrees of regularity, and have prayed with varying degrees of intensity. I've often felt comforted by my connection to God. One thing that has remained consistent: I am a believer and, most importantly, I believe that God is in charge.

Sometimes, Ryder provides me with what is, admittedly, my lame excuse for not attending mass each week. After all, Ryder couldn't possibly sit quietly through a church service, I reason. I guess I just don't believe that I have to be inside a church building for God to hear me and know what's in my heart. My mom definitely does not agree. Thankfully, when TJ was preparing for his First Holy Communion, my mom took him to church every week. She still takes him every single Sunday, confident in the knowledge that at least *she* is ensuring his spot in heaven.

I did go to mass with my parents and TJ on Easter Sunday last year. I watched TJ, perfectly trained by the routine of my mother, recite the *Our Father*. He put his hands together in prayer, fingertips pointed toward the heavens, eyes closed, voice hushed. My recent absence had certainly not dimmed my memory: I put my hands together, fingertips-to-fingertips, and whispered the words of the prayer alongside TJ. At the end of mass, TJ turned to me and said, "You did well your first time, Mom."

"TJ," I answered, "Mommy used to go to church all the time, but now she does the Lord's work at home with your brother." This received an eye roll from my mom.

During the drive home, I expanded on what I said earlier. "TJ, I love that you are enjoying church with Mea every weekend. Remember that each person has his own relationship with God. If you judge people by whether or not they go to mass each week, you are missing what the priest is saying." I gave my mom one of my most pious smiles.

I would be lying if I denied that, at first, it didn't cross my mind that Ryder's diagnosis was punishment for the wrong things I had done in the past. I believe it's normal for people to think this way. I often thought about what I had done to deserve this "punishment." There were periods of my life where I struggled with alcohol. Was it because there were times I drank too much? Or because I said or did some mean things that, if I could, I would turn back the clock and be a kinder, more compassionate person in that moment? Was it because I was selfish? Or spineless? In the end, if we are to believe in God, we have to believe that God is not vengeful. And today, as you know by now, I certainly do not see Ryder's diagnosis as a punishment. Quite the contrary!

Please understand what I am about to say and forgive any unintended sound of narcissism. The journey I have taken with Ryder so far has been enlightening and given me a sense of superiority. This is not superiority over others, but superiority over life itself. I feel that nothing else can hurt me as deeply as my initial hurt with Ryder. I get upset at times, of course, but I am freed from mundane worries.

More than three years after Ryder's diagnosis, I feel much more grateful that autism touched my life so closely than resentful for it. Sometimes I listen to what some people worry about or complain about with their kids and I think, *Really?* I keep one kid in bed with me so I can drape my leg over him just to know he's still in the house during the overnight hours while we try to sleep. The other kid stays in bed with me so that he is reassured that I love him as much as the one I need to leg drape. Who's complaining about the extra carpool drive?

I can't lie, I still have my moments of doubt or disbelief about my fate. Sometimes I turn our corner and I see that "*Autism Child Area*" sign on my block and I wonder, *Wow! How did I get here?* Sometimes I go out to dinner with my small group of local moms, none of whom have a child with autism, and while they're talking, I think about the statistics that we noted earlier as I look around the table and my thoughts drift off. *If it's one in 54 children and one in 45 boys, and together the 6 of us have 17 children, then, I wonder, how many of these other moms were obsessively worried about one of their kids having autism while they were planning a family? Why did my number come up when the heavenly dice were rolled?* And then my attention returns to the table chatter and the enjoyment of friends.

In some ways, my life is a joke on me—in a very good way. How could it not be? Throughout my adult life, I had *one* obsessive fear, strange though it may sound, and that was that I would have a child with autism. And God saw fit that one of my two boys has it. I'm sure you've heard the joke: people make plans and God laughs.

I also believe that a case can be made for some subconscious foreshadowing, that the existence of my fear was actually psychic foreboding; the diagnosis was destined to happen all along. Each of us does have that inner voice. Think about how many times you've said, "*I had a feeling I should have...*" or, "*I knew I was going to...*" The problem, or the issue, is that we often don't acknowledge our inner awareness until well after the fact. Steve Goodier, an author who has written a number of inspirational-type books, wrote about his own journey, "I've learned something along the way: I've learned to heed the call of my heart...I've learned that the voice of fear is not always to be trusted." His words resound for me; remember, I feared having a child with autism well before I was even pregnant. The voice of fear that I heard for so long was definitely not to be trusted. What I feared most, happened, and what happened has opened my mind and my heart. I am blessed by what I feared.

An argument could be made that with all the ABA therapies, Steve and I are hoping to give up the Ry we know, and are trying to conform him, to make him more "normal." I hope against hope that the best of him stays the same, and I hope that we are giving him tools to enable him to succeed in this crazy world. But what if the best of him is *because* of his autism? What if the areas we're hoping to "correct"—with all of these therapies—are exactly the areas that give him his amazing energy and creative perception? If given the opportunity, would I give up the best of him, as he is now, to have him improve socially or emotionally? There are no easy answers.

Most of us have the same dreams when we begin to plan to have a child: we dream of the golden child who stands out because he is healthy, smart, funny, loving, kind, and successful at all that he endeavors. Or at least we want a solidly average son or daughter, who enjoys a solidly excellent life! I think of this and am reminded of all the people who have made headlines because of their *undreamed-of* pitfalls or tragedies, illnesses or accidents. Each was someone's dream child. Despite our world of awareness, acceptance, and tolerance, no one finds out that she's pregnant and hopes that the child will have autism, Down syndrome, be gay or transgender, or anything that people have to come to "accept" or have "awareness" about.

I get angry when my mom suggests that someday we will learn that Ryder has been misdiagnosed, that he doesn't have autism. But then, at the same time, I find wonder if I don't hold the same hopes that my mother has the honesty to *speak*. For example, the other day I had a meeting with Ryder's ABA team and the team leader, Karrie, described Ryder as "textbook Autism," and my heart sank hearing those words out loud. Am I any better than my mom? To be overcome with that sad feelings again as if it's day one of diagnosis and not more than three years in? Am I holding out hope that he'll improve so much that the diagnosis will disappear? Or that he'll not even be recognized as having autism? Am I betraying him when I hold out hope that things can or will change?

I believe that God knows our life's path the day we are born. It's the path that God has set for each of us on the day we were born and that we will follow until the day he calls us home. For the time in between, you can fight against God's will or you can embrace it. I don't know much, but I have learned, despite myself, that internal happiness is found when you embrace it. I have to keep my positivity and my focus on the amazing part of it all, it's what keeps me going: I've been chosen to bear witness to the world's most unjaded human boy grow into manhood. While others may give in to corruption or sin, he, my boy, stays good. He is the best of this world: the heart of it. In that way, to me, he *is* superior to those of us influenced by day-to-day injustices and prejudices. Ryder remains unaware of all that, so he doesn't have to work at staying good. Goodness is just naturally, authentically, Ryder.

When deciding on a title for the book, I realized that there really could only be one. On reflecting on my interaction with Jimmy Muscle over thirty years ago, and assuming that he had a pure heart like that of my son—and I believe he did—it occurred to me how much I had missed out on by not being open to a friendship with him. While I was probably uninterested, ignorant, or scared in my youth, now, as an adult, I have learned—through my son and his friends—to treasure life's unexpected opportunities.

Wouldn't life be boring if everything went according to how we had planned it? Have you ever considered what you are missing out on by not being open to something amazing?

I am sorry Jimmy Muscle, not for picking on you, not for not standing up and defending you when we were kids, but for missing the chance of a friendship between us. For me, you will always be symbolic of a lost opportunity. I'm sorry, Jimmy Muscle. I'm sorry I denied myself the magical joy you most assuredly would have added to my life. If I know you, and I think I now do, you would be happy to know that, in the end, I eventually found that joy.

Afterword

This book was completed when Ryder was in kindergarten. He is now in 5th grade. Thankfully, nowadays, dangerous happenings with him are few and far between. But we never take it for granted. We still helicopter parent him regularly.

CPSIA information can be obtained
at www.ICGtesting.com
Printed in the USA
FSHW011906141120

9 781735 163116